Healing Music

Music

6/50

Healing Music

CAROLYN HUEBNER RANKIN

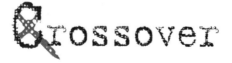

Healing Music

BY: CAROLYN HUEBNER RANKIN

Published by Crossover Publications LLC, 870 N. Bierdeman Road, Pearl, Mississippi 39208, www.crossoverpublications.com
(601) 664-6717, Fax: (601) 664-6818
Randall M. Mooney
Publisher

Library of Congress Control Number: 2010932777

Christian Inspiration
Narrative Non-Fiction

ISBN 978-0-9819657-5-8
Printed in the USA

Cover concept and direction by: DeRanz Graphics & Media, Randall M. Mooney
Cover design and graphic arts by: R. Matthew Mooney

DEDICATION

FOR THE GLORY OF THE LORD JESUS CHRIST
FOR BY HIS STRIPES WE ARE HEALED.

IT IS WITH DEEP APPRECIATION THAT I
DEDICATE THIS BOOK TO MY SURGEONS, KARL
W. SWANN, MD, AND ROBERT G. JOHNSON, MD
OF NEUROSURGICAL ASSOCIATES OF SAN
ANTONIO. TO METHODIST HOSPITAL AND THE
9TH FLOOR STAFF, THEIR OUTSTANDING CARE
AND DEDICATION MADE ALL THE DIFFERENCE IN
MY RECOVERY.

I ALSO WANT TO EXPRESS MY HEARTFELT
APPRECIATION TO GREG M. JACKSON, MD, WHO
HAS CONTINUED TO WALK WITH ME THROUGH
THE JOURNEY OF MY LIFE. HE IS MY FRIEND OF
THE HEART AND THE DOCTOR THAT NEVER GAVE
UP ON ME. DR J, TO YOU MY LOVE AND RESPECT
ALWAYS.

ACKNOWLEDGEMENTS

TO MY HUSBAND JAMES, AND DAUGHTER AUDRA,
FOR THEIR LOVE AND SUPPORT.

TO ROSETTA D. HOESSLI, FOR HER FRIENDSHIP
AND EDITORIAL SKILLS.

TO GIRLFRIEND AND LITTLE BROTHER,
FOR ALWAYS BEING THERE FOR ME.

WITHOUT THEIR EFFORTS, CONTRIBUTIONS AND
PATIENCE, THIS BOOK WOULD
NOT BE POSSIBLE.

BLESSINGS, CAROLYN

Chapter

One

Answer me when I call to you, O my righteous God. Give me relief from my distress; be merciful to me and hear my prayer.

Psalms 4:1

Dr. Paul Hansen studied my x-rays intently, then turned to me and asked, "How old are you, Carolyn?"

I didn't like the look on his face and my heart pounded in my throat. "I turned twenty-eight last month."

Dr. Hansen shook his head and concentrated a few minutes more on the x-rays. Finally, he turned off the viewing box lights and sat down in front of me. "You have degenerative bone disease, Carolyn," he stated without preamble. "Your spine is that of a 90-year-old woman and there's not much we can do for you. The truth is, you'll probably be in a wheelchair by the time you're thirty-five."

He spoke without any emotion, as if he was reciting a lunch menu, but those casually-spoken words ricocheted through my head, bounced off the walls, and made no sense to me. I was the mother of a beautiful two-year-old little girl and the wife of an important executive with a huge oil company. I had an enormous house to run, entertaining to do. There had to be a mistake! I had way too much on my plate for something like this.

I tried to pull myself together and asked the one question I thought might buy me a little time. "Are you sure?"

He nodded. "I've seen this before, Carolyn, but it's usually in people much older than you. You just need to accept this and make plans for your future, because one day you'll go down and never get up again."

I heard his words, but they didn't register. He was a good doctor—he did the physicals for the employees of my husband's company—but he wasn't the only doctor in San Antonio, Texas. After all, we had one of the finest medical communities in the entire country. Desperately ill people came here from all over the world. I could find someone else, another doctor, someone who would say Dr. Hansen was wrong.

Besides, the word *accept* was not in my vocabulary. If I had just *accepted* without a fight everything that life had handed to me over the years, I'd be six feet under by now. I was a fighter by nature. Life had made me that way.

I managed to get to my feet without letting on how much that simple motion hurt. Every muscle and bone in my body screamed out with agony, from my teeth to my toes, but I refused to let it show.

"Thank you very much, Dr. Hansen. May I take these x-rays with me?"

"Certainly; I'm really very sorry, Carolyn."

"Thank you," I repeated automatically, my voice

sounding a million miles away. "I appreciate your help."

Stone-faced, I left his office with my head held high, all 5-feet 2-inches of me cool and controlled. But once outside, I couldn't do it anymore. I surrendered to shock and disbelief and panic. Tears streamed down my face and I could hardly stand up. Finally, shaking all over, I collapsed against the wall and prayed for the strength to drive home.

My short life had been filled with traumatic events, but this was among the worst. It might even be *the* worst. As I pointlessly drove around and around in circles, struggling to find my way out of the parking garage, I remembered how it had all started.

The first time it had happened was in February 1982, the week after my daughter Audra was born. Her birth had been difficult and I had been home from the hospital for just two days, but I was already tidying up the house and taking care of my new bundle of joy. Finally, with my baby asleep and dinner in the oven, I sat down in my chair in the family room, hoping to rest for a few minutes. I closed my eyes and even managed to doze. But when I tried to stand up, I couldn't. I couldn't move my legs.

I called our family doctor right away, but he wasn't too concerned. He knew that I had a tendency to overdo just about everything, so he blamed my situation on the fact that I had had a very long labor and then had probably gone home to pick up my busy life right where I had left it. He prescribed muscle relaxers and pain medication, along with orders to take it easy for awhile.

Tell me, how does a new mother take it easy? I had never known how to do that, and I certainly didn't know how to do it now.

Fortunately, after a few days I returned to my usual routine, but I hadn't been able to shake the feeling that something was very different inside my body. Not *wrong*, exactly, just *different*.

Still, I had diapers to change and bottles to wash, dinner to fix and a house to clean. I was a perfectionist and my priorities were clear. I was so busy that I didn't have a minute to spare, and that's the way I liked it.

By the end of 1982, as if I wasn't busy enough, I had even found the time to fulfill a personal promise I had made to God many years earlier. I began a missing children's organization and named it *Texas Child Search, Inc.* With every ounce of passion I had, I threw myself into my newest labor of love—locating and recovering missing and exploited children. Word of our success had spread like wildfire across the country, and I was busier than ever.

Before long it became clear that I needed help with my growing bundle of energy, so we hired a full-time nanny to take care of her. Leola was a wonderful Christian woman, wise and loving and warm. She was already a grandmother and had many years experience raising children, so I left Audra in her care without a qualm.

In 1985, when Audra was three years old, the morning started like any other morning. My husband Larry left for work, and I piddled around in the kitchen getting Audra's breakfast. Leola was going to be a little late that morning, so I looked forward to spending a bit of extra time alone with Audra.

Breakfast finished, we went into the family room to watch *Sesame Street* on television. Since I liked the program, too, I enjoyed watching it with her whenever I had the chance. Besides, it allowed me to sit down quietly for an hour and think about nothing more serious than Cookie Monster and Big Bird.

But this morning, as soon as I sat down, my dog began barking outside—an insistent, penetrating bark that told me I'd better check it out.

I stood up. And hit the floor. I couldn't move. Excruciating pain, more pain than I had ever experienced in my life, slammed through me and twisted me up like a pretzel.

God, please help me! I've got to get up! I'm alone except for my baby girl and I can't scare her. Oh, God, please help me.

But, after a few minutes of this wrenching agony, I knew I was on my own. I watched my little girl laughing at Cookie Monster and prayed that I would make sense, that she would understand the urgency of what I needed her to do. The phone was out of reach and I was completely helpless. She was just a baby, but she was all I had.

I was amazed at how calm my voice was. "Audra?"

Her laughter stopped and she looked over at me. "You okay, Mommy?"

"I need you to do something very important for me, Audra."

Audra listened very closely to my instructions, attentive in a way she had never been before, and her blue eyes were as round as saucers. When I finished, she just nodded soberly and said, "Okay, Mommy."

Audra got the phone and pushed the button that automatically dialed the number for her daddy's office. When Larry answered, she spoke with great authority. "Daddy, you have to come home right now. Mommy is on the floor and can't get up."

I called out to him so he would know that I was conscious. Then, after she hung up, she went to her room, found her pillow and blanket, dragged them down the stairs, and gently covered me up.

Audra was my little hero at the tender age of three. My husband's office was only five minutes away and he came home immediately. While Larry was shocked to find me like this, Audra took on the role of grown-up, patted me on the head, and said, "You'll be okay, Mommy."

I wasn't at all sure about that, but I tried to nod reassuringly. "Don't worry, sweetheart. I'll be fine."

Yet every time Larry tried to lift me or attempted to move me even slightly, I screamed. I have never felt such pain in my life. The fifty-nine hours of labor I had experienced giving birth to Audra was nothing compared to this pain. This pain brought with it cold sweats and nausea so violent I thought I would pass out. I *prayed* I would pass out. I was sure I was going to die. When Leola finally arrived, she took Audra out of the room so she wouldn't see me cry as Larry moved me towards the couch...inch...by inch...by inch. It took an hour to move me three feet.

Once I was on the couch, Larry called my doctor. An hour later the pharmacy delivered heavy-duty pain medication and muscle relaxers.

I spent the next four days on the couch. Leola took care of me during the day and my husband took care of me during the evening. Even though I was unable to move, I was too stubborn to go to the hospital. I learned to urinate in a bucket and a few other things I needed to know in order to survive life on the couch.

When I was finally able to see our family doctor, he told me that he believed I was suffering from muscle spasms in my lower back. "They can make you miserable, Carolyn," he explained, as if I didn't know that. "They really hurt. I want you to stay on the muscle relaxants and pain meds every day for awhile and we'll see how you do."

Even without my doctor's prodding, I knew I needed to slow down a little, and I really did try, but I just didn't know how to do that. I've always had to stay busy. So I returned to my life, living in some sort of rosy-hued state of denial, and prayed that I wouldn't ever go through that kind of pain again.

The following Sunday was Easter, and I had invited our neighbor over for dinner. Mr. Castro was a lonely old man, a recent widower, and he was really looking forward to a good home-cooked meal. Since one of my favorite things to do is to entertain and take care of folks, I was busy setting the dining room table. The ham was in the oven, the sweet potatoes were keeping warm, and the house smelled wonderful. After I had checked the oven one last time, I turned toward the dining room—and the pain shot through my legs. I grabbed the chair and counter to steady myself.

Oh, no, not again...not today.

I was determined not to spend the next week on the floor, so I managed to make it around to the side of my kitchen where there's a narrow, steep staircase with a good handrail leading up to the foyer of our second floor. With a Herculean effort I pulled myself up those steps and made it to the top, then managed to get to my bedroom and onto the bed. Easter dinner was a covered plate that my husband took over to poor old Mr. Castro, with my abject apologies.

After another week in bed I knew it was time to see a different doctor, someone more specialized, and so I had gone to see Dr. Paul Hansen.

Now, as I drove from his office to my home, I kept asking, over and over: *Dear God, what is happening to me? Why this? Why me?*

Well, at least I finally knew the answer to that question, if not the reason. Dr. Hansen had given me a diagnosis. In my mind's eye, I saw those three words in capital letters, DEGENERATIVE BONE DISEASE, and I understood. Those three words were going to end my life as I knew it.

Chapter Two

I sign now my defense—let the Almighty answer me...

Job 31:35

I'm no different from the rest of the human race. If you give me bad news and I don't want to hear it, I'll put you on the back burner until I can handle what you have to say. However, the problem with this attitude, especially as it relates to medical issues, is that it keeps you from doing what you need to do as soon as you need to do it.

Yet that had always been my way. I could put off, or hide from, anything if it made me uncomfortable enough. But this time was different. This time I knew I had to handle this situation as soon as I possibly could.

This time my response was to make an appointment with Dr. Albert Sanders, an orthopedic specialist who had been recommended to me by a friend whose father was a prominent attorney in San Antonio and who knew all the best doctors. What he had to say was far more palatable than anything I had heard from Dr. Hansen.

"Yes, you have degenerative bone disease, Carolyn," he said, closely studying my x-rays on his viewing box, "and, yes, your spine looks pretty awful, but I think we can manage this for awhile."

I was so thrilled that my heart literally skipped a beat or two. "Really?"

"I think so. We need to keep you moving, and we need to manage the pain effectively. Let's try it this way."

Dr. Sanders' first order was to fit me with a custom-made back brace that would support my lower spine. It turned out to be a corset-type garment with two steel rods in the back that I could wear under loose-fitting clothes. I wasn't too thrilled with it; after all—I was a young woman with a certain amount of vanity. But I have to admit, it was the answer to a prayer whenever that insidious but undeniable weakness began to creep into my legs. When that happened, I girded myself up in the brace and was able to avoid the floor.

While Dr. Sanders tried hard to keep me upbeat and optimistic, he didn't mince words, either. "You *have* to change your lifestyle, Carolyn," he told me emphatically. "You have to think through everything you do before you do it. Ask yourself: Can this activity hurt me? If you can see a way that it could, keep in mind that what might only strain a normal person could well paralyze you. Ask yourself if you're willing to risk that before you take on any kind of activity. Also, keep in mind that if you go somewhere alone, you might have an episode that would cause you to be dependent on people you don't know to take care of you. I don't know how you feel about that, but you need to be aware of that possibility."

At least Dr. Sanders didn't say I would be in a wheelchair by the time I was 35. I would do just about anything to keep that image at bay, including turning my whole life upside down.

But still, as the pain came and went in debilitating waves and my legs seemed to grow weaker with the passage of time, I kept asking: Why me, God? Why is this happening to me?

I learned that the oft-recited adage, *you don't have anything if you don't have your health*, is absolutely true. If an outsider looked in at my life, my life would have appeared perfect. My husband made an excellent living and seemed to dote on his family. My little girl was beautiful and smart and full of personality. My organization was running full-throttle and making a difference in the lives of many despairing families. I, it seemed, had everything my heart could possibly desire. What else, an outsider would ask, could God give you that you don't already have?

To those of you reading this, the obvious answer would be the healing of my gradually disintegrating bones. But the truth is I needed much more than that. The physical pain caused by my collapsing spine actually masked a deeper emotional pain that I had run from for years, and it was pain that God would soon force me to face head-on.

The Bible is filled with stories of miracle healings, and I had learned those stories at the knee of my devoutly Christian father who had raised me in the Assembly of God Church. Now, not surprisingly considering the circumstances, I remembered those stories and wondered if they could possibly pertain to me.

As quickly as that thought came to me, I put it back into

mothballs—where all my spiritual thoughts had pretty much been placed over the last decade or so. I was sure that God didn't have time for a person like me, and He certainly wouldn't hear a prayer uttered from the lips of someone as sinful as I was. I was disgusted with myself when I realized that I, like everyone else, didn't reach out to God until I was in trouble, and I didn't want to be a person like that.

On the other hand, I wasn't above a little self-pity. In fact, if I tell the full truth, I wasn't above a whole lot of self-pity. *How could this happen to me? Haven't I suffered enough in my life already?*

I won't go into the trauma of my childhood or the repercussions of it—that's an entirely different book and one that I've already written. But I will say that probably the most difficult thing I've ever gone through in my life was the death of my father when I was just fifteen years old.

When my daddy died, I had no reason to go on living. That's not an emotional statement; it's the truth. Then, I guess because they didn't want to deal with me for a variety of reasons, my family sent me out to relatives I barely knew in California, which was about as far away from my little hometown of White Oak, Pennsylvania as they could get. While all this was difficult for me to handle at such a young age, it did help me to develop persistence, determination, and an ability to move beyond challenges.

It also created in me a desperate need to be perfect. If I was perfect, people would love me. If I was perfect, people would look up to me. They would want to *be* me. If I was perfect on the outside, then no one would know how worthless and unlovable I was on the inside.

With all this confusion and turbulence banging around in my spirit, it's no wonder that I drifted for a number of years before I finally made my way to Houston, Texas. I met Larry there and married him in 1978, for all the wrong reasons. But at least I had a family again and a reason to live—at the ripe old age of twenty.

When Larry was transferred to San Antonio and we moved into a beautiful old home I had literally seen in my dreams for many years, I became aware of another emotion I had never been aware of before: *anger*. I was angry with everyone. I was angry with people in my past, people in my present, and people I hadn't even met yet. I was cynical, defensive, and prepared to justify everything I did, right or wrong.

But most of all, I was angry with God. He had taken my daddy—how could He do such a thing to me? Didn't He realize that I needed my father down here on earth with me more than He needed him up there in Heaven? He had pulled me from the warmth of my family and tossed me defenseless into a world that chewed children up and spit them out. What had He been thinking? What had I done so awful that He felt the need to take so much from me?

If self-pity was my first name, anger was my second. But at least I was still *talking* to God, even if I was chewing Him out most of the time. I don't think I was ever in a place that I wasn't aware of His Presence in my life.

Finally, as the years passed and motherhood matured me, my anger towards God gradually subsided and I was able to converse with Him a little more civilly than before, that is until I was diagnosed with this bone disease. Then I went beyond anger. I was beside myself. I was outraged at what I saw as the unfairness of my life.

While I'm embarrassed to even admit that, I also have to say that I believe my anger was the fuel that kept me motivated. In my typically strong-willed, bring-it-on manner, I refused to give up my battle to defeat what I saw as the monster that now dominated my world.

In addition to this ongoing personal struggle, I had an angry and frustrated husband to deal with as well. Quite often, when I didn't feel up to going with him somewhere or didn't want to do something he wanted to do, his solution was to get mad, throw a few curse words my way, storm out with Audra and leave me home alone. While I was truly sorry, I was much sorrier about how my disease affected my daughter than about how it affected my husband. He was a grown man and he should have understood my limitations, but it was Audra that my heart really ached for.

My little girl was growing up and I wanted to do so much with her. Whenever I felt well enough, we went out and tried to do normal 'mom-and-daughter' things together. But there were limits to what I could do. I couldn't walk long distances—I could hardly walk the mall anymore, so hiking was out. I couldn't sit for extended periods of time, but I couldn't stand, either. My dreams of taking her to the zoo, or a children's museum, or a park playground went into the shadows of what had once been the activities of my life. Pain became my nearly constant companion.

Through it all, Audra seemed to understand that her mommy had a problem and that we really just needed to stay at home. She never seemed to hold it against me the way her father did, and I was so grateful for that. We watched her favorite movies and read books together in bed. We colored and made up stories, and popcorn was always handy.

Audra seemed to be content with the fact that I couldn't do much, and when I look back on it, I understand that she probably was. She had my undivided attention at those times, and children don't need much more than that. When I was well, I worked frantically to stay caught up for when the next 'down' time came, and Audra was usually shuttled to the background while I did everything else I thought I was supposed to do. But when I was sick, I was forced to be still, and I was hers.

In 1991 we borrowed a friend's small travel trailer and headed back east to see my family and friends. It was the first vacation we had taken together in years and I couldn't wait to go, even though I had just recovered from a month-long bout with paralysis and was still just barely walking with a cane. Still, I managed to pack the trailer with all we needed for such a long trip, and I managed to do it without letting on how much pain I was in.

The first leg of our journey ended in White Oak, Pennsylvania, the little town in which I had been raised, and where my mother, sister and brother still lived. Although my memories of the last time I had been here were unpleasant to say the least, it was still nice to be back and see all the familiar places I had loved as a child.

As we drove up to my mother's home, we passed the Rankin farmhouse—a quaint and picturesque dwelling that had meant so much to me when I was struggling through the nightmares of my childhood and early adolescence. I was shocked when nostalgic tears actually burned my eyes.

I turned my face away so Larry couldn't see my emotion. "I need to visit Grandma Rankin. She meant so much to me when I was little."

Larry shrugged and yawned. "You can visit anyone you want."

I ignored his indifference and kept talking, remembering. "She was like my own grandmother, you know what I mean? She taught me so much. To this day I crochet the way she taught me…and, well, she even taught me to grow African Violets like the ones I have on the window sill in the kitchen."

Larry yawned again and nodded. "I know, Carolyn, I know. You go on and visit her."

I looked at him and shook my head. The man had absolutely no passion; nothing ever seemed to truly touch him. Every once in awhile I envied him that detachment, but most of the time I felt sorry for him—and I felt sorry for him now. He would never know how it felt to love someone the way I still loved Grandma Rankin.

I could envision that old woman at that moment as clearly as if I had just seen her yesterday. She was feisty and opinionated, with beautiful silver hair, cornflower blue eyes, and a dazzling smile that radiated joy and peace. Her husband had died back in the '60s, and her two sons were grown with families of their own. Even though her family lived nearby, she seemed to spend a lot of time alone with only her dachshund, Heinzy, to keep her company.

I had loved the hours I spent with her because she never made me feel like I was in the way. She was never in a hurry; she was the most patient person I ever knew. But what I remembered most about her was that she felt a love for the Lord that would shake the foundations of her old two-story farmhouse. As we cooked, or crocheted, or piddled in the garden, she told me stories about her life and how Jesus was the answer to all of our troubles. And even when I doubted that, which was often, she had me believing it by the end of the day. Her faith was open and contagious, even to a child struggling with demons and memories that were beyond human understanding. Her Bible was always open nearby, and she could quote scripture better than any preacher I ever heard.

Now, as we drove toward my mother's house, I felt the warm stirrings of experiences long past and long forgotten: my early years singing in the children's choir at church, my pride when I watched my parents' baptism, my father's gentle voice when we prayed together at night. The peaceful, spiritual part of my life had been lost in the frenetic pace of my daily routine; I had squandered it on my anger and self-pity. Now, more than anything, I realized that I needed to find it again.

Chapter
Three

O my Lord, I take refuge in you; save
and deliver me from all who pursue
me, or they will tear me to pieces
like a lion and rip me to pieces
with no one to rescue me.

Psalms 7:1

"Larry, do you want to come with me to visit Grandma Rankin?"

I set my basket of laundry down on the sofa and waited for his answer, but his gaze was glued to some college football game on television. He shook his head in irritation and waved me off. "Go ahead. Have fun."

"Well, Audra's with Mom, so you'll have the whole afternoon to yourself. I'll see you later."

After I had put away our laundry, I called Grandma Rankin's house. It was amazing that I could still remember her phone number after all these years, but it returned to me so easily that I wondered if it hadn't always been there, just waiting for me to summon it.

A deep voice answered, one that I didn't recognize, and I wondered if I had dialed the wrong number after all. "Is this Viola Rankin's residence?" I asked.

"Yes, it is."

I frowned. "Can I ask who this is?"

"This is Jim."

I couldn't believe it. *Little Jimmy Rankin.* I hadn't seen him since I was 15 years old, back in 1973.

"Oh...my...gosh. Little Jimmy Rankin. Is that really you?"

He was clearly puzzled. "It's really me. Who's this?"

"Take a guess. I used to be your best friend."

There was a long, silent pause. "Carolyn," he said finally. "Carolyn Sue Shaw."

"It's me. What are you doing there?"

"I live here with Grandma. Where are you?"

"I'm at my mom's house. Can I come see you and Grandma right now?"

There was no denying the anticipation in his voice. "Come on down! I'll be right here waiting for you. Hurry up!"

I shared his excitement. It had been years since I had set my eyes on him, but it hadn't even occurred to me that I would get to see him this trip. He had lived just a few houses down from me when we were kids and we were best friends until the day I left home. He was what the kids today call a 'nerd' because he was extremely smart, loved to read, and preferred to fantasize about space travel rather than joining the other children in some neighborhood game. In fact, I had once told my father that I was going to marry little Jimmy Rankin when I grew up because I was sure nobody else would.

Using my cane, I walked slowly to the truck, frustrated because I couldn't get into the driver's seat any faster than this snail's pace and get down the hill.

As I pulled up to the massive, still-majestic landmark farmhouse, my heart filled to overflowing with loving memories of the men and women who had, through many generations, lived in this place. The Rankin family, tough Scottish pioneers who had settled in our part of western Pennsylvania after the Revolutionary War, once owned all the land where the homes in our neighborhood were now located. Towns, counties and roads had been named in their honor.

Now, as if the Rankins I had known were all still breathing and standing in front of me, I saw now-deceased Ross, Ed, Aunt Olive, Aunt Bell and Abbey—the very people who had filled this land with vineyards and apple orchards; treasures from my childhood.

I put the truck in park, turned off the engine, and turned my gaze toward a huge old cast-iron bell near the house. That bell had weathered hundreds of winters standing on its post like a sentinel at its station. Every time Aunt Olive would let me, I rang that bell, feeling very important, to call the men in from the fields for lunch. Swinging from that rope, I gave it all I had until she told me to stop.

A movement from the front porch caught my eye and I did a double-take in complete disbelief. Standing beside the door was a great big man with a shock of deep auburn hair—I don't know how else to describe him. I managed to get out of my truck without letting on how wracked with pain I was and made my way slowly to the porch. Leaning on my cane, I walked over to the back door and stood in front of him, my gaze traveling slowly from his chest to the top of his head.

It took me awhile to find my voice. And when I did, all I could do was blurt, "My God, Jimmy, you're so handsome!"

He smiled and opened the door for me. Once I was inside the house, I turned and gave him a hug.

"And big," I added.

He grinned. "I've always been big. You just don't remember."

Well, he might have been big, I thought ruefully, but he certainly hadn't been handsome. He had been a tall, chunky kid who liked to take imaginary space trips in boxes that he had turned into rocket ships—nothing special.

Well, he was sure special now. Now he took my breath away. I followed him into the dining room and stood there silently for a long moment, soaking in the memories. That great table held hundreds of recollections for me in the same way that the big claw-footed hutch held the family china. Out of the corner of my eye I saw the ghost of a blonde, blue-eyed little girl sitting on a stack of telephone books, eating lunch with the family. She was so real I smiled at her.

I followed Jim from the dining room, made my way past the grand staircase, and entered the parlor. There on the sofa, her welcoming arms opened wide, was Grandma Rankin. Her silver hair framed her face and her creamy complexion bore not a hint that she had spent 90 years on this earth. I shrieked with joy and fell into her embrace, burying my face in her ample breast.

I could have stayed there forever, but Grandma Rankin was having none of it. "Get up, child!" she ordered. "Let me look at you!"

I got to my feet carefully then sat next to her, holding her hand in mine. Jimmy sat across from us, an old guitar leaning against his chair, and we had so much to say to each other that we all seemed to be talking at once. Finally, after we had covered the local gossip and our conversation was finally running down, Grandma Rankin looked at me closely and asked, "Carolyn, why are you using that cane?"

I didn't want to go into it and shook my head, but her fingers tightened around mine with surprising strength. I gave in instantly. I had no choice. I knew that if Grandma Rankin asked me a direct question, I'd better give her a direct answer and quick.

I made one last attempt. "Please, Grandma. I don't want to waste our time together."

"I've got all the time in the world, child," she interrupted. "Why the cane?"

I looked at Jimmy imploringly, but his eyes told me he wanted the answer, too. I knew then that there was no alternative.

As I described the dreaded bone disease that had come to rule my daily life, a sense of true apprehension filled the room. For the first time, I realized that I hadn't shared my anguish and fear with anyone who really knew me and really cared. I had close friends back home that I usually told everything going on in my life, of course, but I hadn't told them about this. I didn't want anyone to feel sorry for me. Good health, vitality and strength were important to my work with both law enforcement and traumatized families, so I had kept this situation to myself. It was dangerous to let the word out.

Now I realized what a tremendous relief it was to talk about my fear, how much pain I was in, and even about my loneliness. Most people don't want to listen to stories like mine, but Jimmy and Grandma Rankin listened intently to everything I said. Finally I just ran out of words, slowly, like a well-conditioned athlete runs out of energy, and Grandma Rankin patted my hand.

"It'll be all right, child. You'll see."

I didn't understand where her conviction came from, but I nodded as if I did. I smiled. "Can we talk about something else? I didn't come over here to moan and groan all day. I'm really sorry."

"Of course," she answered, patting my hand again. "Play us something, Jimmy."

When Jimmy picked up that guitar and strummed a few opening chords, I closed my eyes and snuggled closer to the elderly woman beside me. I have always been moved by music, but this music was special, different. It didn't feel like it was of this world, but instead as if Jimmy was tapping in to some other dimension when he played. The simplicity of the songs he sang about his love for the Lord enveloped me in a kind of velvet serenity, soothing my spirit and easing my fear. His voice was beautiful and I could have listened for days.

Finally, as much as I hated to, I had to leave. I had only planned to visit for 30 minutes, yet hours had flown by. But what a treat it had been!

"I have to get back home now," I said finally. "I have laundry to finish and supper to start." Tears pricked my eyes and I had to take a moment to compose myself before I added, "But it's been wonderful seeing you both! I've missed you so much."

"Carolyn...Wait." Jimmy's deep voice trailed away uncertainly.

"Yes?"

"Carolyn, let us pray for you that the Lord touch your back in a mighty way."

I looked at him, frowning, then said to myself: *Well, why not?*

It wasn't that I didn't believe the Lord *could* touch my back 'in a mighty way,' but that I didn't know why He would bother. I couldn't even count all the times I had lied, felt sorry for myself, lost my temper, wanted something that belonged to somebody else, taken His name in vain and even cried out against Him in anger.

The list of sins I had committed in my lifetime was endless. I was absolutely positive that God would not give me a moment's notice when there were so many more important matters in this world demanding His attention.

Still, as Jimmy stood up and placed his hand on my shoulder, the look in his eyes was mesmerizing, commanding, as if he *had* to pray for me. I couldn't look away from him, and I couldn't refuse. I moved closer to Grandma on the sofa and she held my hand more tightly than ever; Jimmy sat next to me and placed his hand on my lower back. I closed my eyes and bowed my head.

Jimmy began to pray in a voice so low I could hardly hear him. After a few moments Grandma Rankin joined him in prayer, softly at first, then louder, until their voices swelled as they cried out words I couldn't comprehend. With an intensity I had never heard before, their shouts went up to heaven as they pleaded with Jesus to touch me, to heal me, to deliver me from this wretched condition. And although I couldn't understand what they were saying, I knew that God could.

Heat radiated from both Jimmy and Grandma and surged into my body, filling my soul and somehow easing my pain. Tears of joy streamed like rivers down my face as I felt the love of God flow into the room and gradually envelop me in warmth and peace.

Was God really doing this for me?

Finally their voices dropped into whispers and the prayer was finished. I lifted my head, opened my eyes, and looked around the parlor, expecting to see something mystical somewhere, like a radiant light or beautiful colors. But the room hadn't changed.

Only I had.

Grandma Rankin kissed my cheek. "Trust in Jesus, child. He'll take care of you."

Trust in Jesus, I thought. After all the years I had been so angry with God, could I really do that now? Wasn't it too late? Could He really still care about me? Then, as I remembered the warmth of God's love surging through that parlor like a tidal wave, I reminded myself that His love passed all human understanding.

I gripped my cane to steady myself and stood up carefully, waiting until I had my balance before I took a step away from the sofa. I held my hand down to Grandma and helped her to her feet, then took her in my arms.

"I love you, Grandma," I whispered in her ear. "I truly love you."

"I love you, too, child."

Jimmy walked with me to the truck and opened the door, then kissed me gently on the cheek. Tears rolled down my face as I put my cane inside and climbed up into the seat. Through the open window I held Jimmy's hand and managed to smile. As I met his gaze, I was surprised to see that his eyes were swimming with tears as well.

How could this be happening? This handsome man who had been the chubby red-headed boy I walked with to the bus stop each day, who had given me my first kiss, the boy I told my daddy I would marry when I grew up. How could he have tears for me?

I never wanted to let go of his hand, but I finally did. As I backed the truck out of the drive and turned onto the street, little Jimmy Rankin remained in sight, still waving, until I turned the corner. He disappeared from view.

Something wonderful had happened to me, but I wasn't sure what it was. Yet I was sure about one thing: I was forever altered.

𝄞

Our summer vacation over, life returned to normal. Audra went back to school and our routine became manageable again. It wouldn't be long before autumn winds finally blustered into the city and people would venture from their air-conditioned homes to enjoy the coolness, work in their yards or talk with their neighbors.

I continued to maintain a careful lifestyle. I tried to get enough rest whenever I could and I took my medications religiously to ward off the advancing effects of my bone disease. My regular physician, Dr. Greg Jackson (I fondly nicknamed him *Dr. J*) was always available to me and had become more than just my doctor. He also became my friend and my unflagging supporter. To this day, I don't know what I would do without him.

I started to lose feeling in my legs and I stumbled a lot. I noticed, too, that sometimes my left foot drooped slightly. Finally, concerned, Dr. J set an appointment for me to see Dr. James Story, Chief of Neurology at the Texas Medical University. Dr. Story was a tall, burly man who could have been very intimidating had he not been so gentle. He put me through a series of tests that analyzed my motor skills, then took a sharp object and ran it over my legs. Sometimes I would feel it, sometimes I couldn't.

It was clear that I wasn't winning this battle. Dr. Story looked closely at the MRI of my spine. "Carolyn, the nerves to your legs are being affected by the condition of your lumbar spine. I don't think there's much we can do to correct the pressure on your nerves except to continue with good pain management. What you do need to know, though, is that not only are your legs going to continue to be affected, but you may begin to have problems with bladder and bowel control as well."

Great, I thought in disgust, visualizing enormous diapers looming right above my horizon. What a future. But I had two wonderful doctors who intended to keep that from happening if there was any way they could, and they worked closely together to keep me functioning and comfortable. I remained on a regimen of drug therapy that didn't include any opiates, since I was very sensitive to different medications, so I was able to stay busy and productive.

As the years rolled by, I kept my fingers crossed. I hadn't suffered any major paralysis episodes since 1991. Was it because I was being such a good girl and doing everything I was told, I wondered, or was it the prayer at the Rankin farmhouse? I didn't know. But whatever the reason, I was grateful.

Chapter Four

A father to the fatherless, a defender of widows is God in His holy dwelling, God sets the lonely in families...

Psalms 68:5, 6

It was 1994 and I ordered a new Chevy Suburban 2500. This vehicle had an all leather interior with a TV/video player in the backseat for Audra, and was tricked out with a telephone and fuzz buster. But it also came with something else: a Bruno lift in the rear for my newly purchased electric scooter.

The day had finally come that if I was going to travel any distance, I had to do it on the scooter. I was now officially handicapped, with parking privileges in all the best places at the mall. My scooter was candy apple red with a basket on the front. If this was my destiny, I wanted to look like I was enjoying it.

My new Suburban and my little red scooter allowed me to keep some of my independence and self-respect. That was so important to me. At least I could go shopping at the mall all by myself, and, although I was an expert shopper, shopping on a scooter was a whole new adventure for me.

Store aisles are often blocked with sale items, and I held my breath as I squeaked by, praying not to knock the whole thing over as I passed. I had to learn to navigate my way in and out of automatic and non-automatic doors, which is a challenge beyond description. I discovered that my view of the world from the seat of a scooter was much different than I imagined. I was basically at the level of a seven-year-old and that would have been okay if I was seven years old, but I was thirty-six. Well, what can I say? I had to deal with it.

Most of the time people are kind, even eager to help you navigate the stores. They see you on the scooter and immediately know that 'something is wrong' with you. Often a sympathetic smile comes your way and that's fine. But, other times, folks have a way of looking *through* you, as if they're afraid to look you in the eye in case your dreadful condition might get passed on to them.

Children are the best. They can't take their eyes off you when you're riding a scooter chair. They're captivated by the fact that you're getting to ride this neat thing and they think it has to be fun. I always smiled at the children—especially when a parent was dragging them along, ordering them not to stare.

Kids are naturally curious about anything that's different from what they think is 'normal.' I've even offered to take children for a ride just to let them know that I was okay with their interest. Parents should let their youngsters look and understand the plight of handicapped people, no matter how minor or severe the handicap may be. If you teach your children to have compassion for others when they're young, acceptance and tolerance will grow and mature along with them.

The Suburban and my scooter became vital extensions of my legs. Maybe I had a false sense of security, but they helped me feel better about the changes in my life. I held on to my independence with a mighty grip, daring anyone to try to pry my fingers loose from the wheel. I had the phone, so I could get help if I needed it, but I would only use it as a last resort.

Still, my life was shrinking and I knew it. Everywhere I went was measured by my access to that scooter. Some days I felt I could walk the distance, other days I had to use the scooter, but the bottom line was this: I had passed my landmark age of thirty-five and I was still moving.

♪

I think it was John Lennon who sang about life being what happens when we're busy making other plans, but whoever it was, he (or she) was absolutely right.

I thought 1994 was going to be an uneventful year in my life. Larry and I were actually learning to get along like old married people, and my little red scooter accompanied us everywhere we went. Larry didn't lose his temper as easily over issues I couldn't change, and I tried to be more tolerant of him as well. Audra was growing into a lovely young lady and we were both very proud of her. Our little family had become a fairly peaceful unit.

We purchased a travel trailer of our own in 1994 and used our new Suburban to tow it as we set off on another vacation that summer to Branson, Missouri. Located in the gorgeous Ozark Mountains, Branson is a perfect vacation spot for a young family, offering everything from fishing, hunting, and water sports to antiquing, collectible shopping, and fabulous entertainment. Even the hot August temperatures, so miserable in San Antonio, are pleasant in the Ozarks.

My favorite place was *Silver Dollar City*, one of the main attractions in the Branson area. The minute I entered its gates, I was transported back a century earlier when the Ozark craftsmen built and sold their wares in the community. Here they created leather goods, blown glass, wood carving, painting, quilting and so much more, just as they had a hundred years before. As I motored up and down the streets of the city on my little scooter, laughing and loving my independence, it was easy to forget we lived in the 20th Century. It was also easy to forget that I was almost completely dependent on that little red scooter.

I believed this family vacation was our best ever. Little did I know it would also be our last. Larry died of a massive heart attack two months later.

$\oint$

Now thirty-six years old, I was widowed with a daughter and disabled. I have to admit I didn't handle it very well. My anger with God returned full throttle, and when I wasn't mad I couldn't stop crying. Life was so unfair I didn't know if I wanted to go on.

Finally, near Christmastime, I decided to take Audra on a trip back east. I knew we would ultimately spend some time with my family in White Oak, Pennsylvania, but I didn't want to be with them at Christmas. My mother wasn't a warm woman, to put it mildly, and my sister, a widow herself for many years, would do nothing but yammer in my ear about how I should live the rest of my life. I just wasn't up to that.

I decided instead to spend Christmas at Virginia Beach, Virginia, in the famous *Founder's Inn*. There, people I didn't know welcomed us into their Christmas celebrations and shared their love for Jesus with us. It was as nice as it could be, considering.

A few days after Christmas, we drove up to Pennsylvania, stopping overnight at my brother's mountain lake house before we headed on into White Oak. I was numb, detached. I looked over at my little girl, hoping that her sweet face would make me feel something. And it did. It made me feel ashamed.

As if she could read my mind, Audra asked quietly, "Mommy, when are you going to stop crying?"

That was when I knew it was time. I had to pull myself together.

$\oint$

My mother and I hadn't been close for years and I didn't expect much from her during my visit. Still, it was good to be in my old bedroom, even if it no longer looked the same. Now it only contained two twin beds and a dresser, but Audra and I didn't need any more than that. I had no agenda and there was nowhere I needed to be. No place felt right for me. I was a foreigner in my own world.

News of Larry's death traveled fast among my family and friends in White Oak. I received a few calls of condolence, but that was all. I had discovered years earlier that people usually don't know what to say during a crisis, so I didn't blame folks for not calling. Besides, I hadn't lived in White Oak for so long that I really didn't have any close friends there anymore. I had left all my real friends back in Texas.

I began to regret my trip back east.

Then Jimmy Rankin called and asked if he could take me to dinner. The whole dating scene frightened me after having been married for so long, but Jimmy was different. He wasn't a stranger. In fact, we had written each other a couple of letters a year since our reunion in 1991, so I knew our feelings were still pretty strong.

I decided to take the plunge. "Well, Jimmy, if I'm going out on my first date in years, I might as well go out with someone I've known my whole life."

Audra was thrilled and ran to our room to see what I could wear on my date. She hollered downstairs, "C'mon, Mom! You have to get ready!"

Jimmy and I had dinner at a restaurant that had been popular when we were kids. He looked a bit nervous and I felt like I was covered in flashing neon lights that read: Disabled Widow on the Dating Scene.

Stop this, Carolyn. You've got to get a grip. Jimmy's an old friend and a Christian gentleman. Relax and enjoy the evening.

So I did.

How our relationship flourished is a book in itself and I might one day write it, but it's the end result that matters now. I learned that the Lord does move in mysterious ways and His ways are not our ways, but He will give you the desires of your heart if you trust Him.

Jimmy Rankin gave up his home, job and inheritance, and moved to Texas. We married in 1998. When I met Jimmy at the altar in our church, there was nowhere else I wanted to be. I wanted to stand with the man I loved before God and witnesses who were my friends. My beautiful teen-aged daughter Audra was my maid of honor. She was so happy you would have thought it was *her* wedding. And, in a way, it was.

I always nickname people I care about, so I called Jim *Rank*, along with a few other sweet names that will remain private. After all, 'Jimmy' had been a red-haired, fair-skinned boy I knew when I was a kid, not this big handsome man who was now my husband, so I had to give him a more adult name. Audra called him *Daddy* from the very earliest days of our marriage, and that's exactly what he is to her. A few years later, upon her request, Jim legally adopted her and we were officially a family.

Life was good. I never thought marriage could be so wonderful, but it was Jim's relationship with the Lord that made him special. The only other real Christian man in my life had been my father, and he'd been gone a long time. But I recognized the same peace and love that had filled my dad also filled my husband.

I continued to have small episodes that put me in bed for a day or two, but nothing like before. Stress had always affected my condition, and my life was now much less stressful. Still, pain was always in the background of my life. Jim prayed for me daily and this gave me great comfort.

In fact, I would actually say this: Husbands, pray for and over your wives daily. This is the greatest act of love you can do for them, to hold them up before the throne of God.

Jim became a high school science teacher, teaching Human Anatomy and Physiology. He had planned to become a doctor, but a series of interruptions kept him from finishing college in Pennsylvania. Once in Texas he thought about returning to medical school but changed his mind. He obtained his teacher's certification instead and today is very happy preparing senior high school students for a possible future in the field of medicine. His 'kids' call him *Dr. Rankin* and he runs his classroom like a mini-medical school.

In the fall of 1999, walking became difficult. The nerves in my legs sent out the wrong signals or no signals at all, so I had to use my walker to get around. Finally, desperate and frightened, I visited my rheumatologist. He suggested I try Vioxx, a new drug that seemed to help many of his patients.

Vioxx changed my life. After only two days, I climbed out of bed and felt my feet touch the floor. I had lost most of the feeling in my feet and thought I would never recover it again. For years, if I had banged or cut my legs or feet, I didn't even know until I saw blood or bruises. Now I could feel my feet again. Overjoyed, I called my doctor and gave him the good news.

After several months I began to feel more like my old self. My pain had lessened and I could walk further without resorting to the scooter. Knowing that I was feeling better made all the difference in Audra. She realized she could go out and not worry about leaving me alone. Rank took such good care of me that she felt I didn't need her anymore. Well, I still needed her, but my husband made his family a priority and nothing came before our health and safety. Audra knew she could leave me in his care, so she began to live a more normal teenage life.

Thank you, Lord, for easing the burden for my little girl.

With the new hope and comfort that Vioxx gave me, I was able to live life much more abundantly. In the summers we traveled the United States in our RV; I wanted to see it all. We visited the Grand Canyon, Mount Rushmore, Montana, Wyoming, Colorado, California and Nevada—just to name a few places.

In November 2000, I retired the Suburban as our main tow vehicle and bought a custom Ford 550 hauler with a low profile bed, designed especially for towing a fifth-wheel trailer.

The truck was decked out with extra fuel tanks and air ride, all leather interior, and special lighting on the outside. We were living large and loving it. But I had the Bruno lift installed on the Ford for my cherry red scooter, just in case.

For Christmas 2001, we drove to California to spend the holiday with some of my old friends in the southern desert of the state. Then, on December 28th, we traveled on to Nevada to spend New Year's Eve in Las Vegas, where the largest display of fireworks in history would occur.

On our way to Las Vegas, we put in at Primm, Nevada. It was actually an area that had three casino/resorts and an RV Park. This was a good place to hang out for two days until our reservations at *Circus Circus* in Las Vegas became effective on the 30th.

Or so we thought....

Chapter Five

Then I heard the voice of the Lord saying, "Whom shall I send? And who will go for us?" And I said, "Here I am. Send me!"

Isaiah 6:8

In the RV park at Primm Valley, we listened to a roller coaster located at the nearby *Buffalo Bill's Casino*. It roared around and around the property, all day and half the night, and actually seemed to vanish *inside* the casino. Jim and I had been watching this monstrosity through our window and I was curious about how it worked. My coaster days were over and I didn't want to ride it. I just wanted to see it up close. Audra decided to stay in the rig and watch a movie, so after dinner Jim and I ventured over to Buffalo Bill's on our own.

Buffalo Bill's Casino has an 1880's mining camp theme and there was so much stuff hanging from the ceilings and walls that we could hardly find the roller coaster area. We were only inside for about thirty minutes when I'd had enough of the noise, color and lights, but the casino—like all casinos had made it nearly impossible for us to leave. It took us forever just to find an *exit* sign.

Finally we stopped at the end of an aisle intersecting with the main walkway, trying to get our bearings. Suddenly a man flew out from nowhere and slammed into me with such force that I crashed backward into Jim. The wind was knocked completely out of me and I literally saw stars. The man swore and kept running.

"Carolyn, are you all right?" Jim asked anxiously, beginning to check me out.

I shook my head. I knew I wasn't. Once security had been notified, we were escorted into a private area. The security chief, who was also an EMT, asked what happened. I told him how I had been bulldozed by the man and gave his description.

The chief nodded, "I know him. He's an employee here."

All I could do was stare at him, stunned. Why wouldn't an employee have stopped to help after knocking over a customer? This guy had sworn at me and taken off like a bat out of… well, you get the picture.

My injuries ranged from a broken right lower molar and a jaw that didn't feel like it lined up anymore. We were fifty miles from a hospital, way too far for me to leave Audra alone, and besides, I could still walk. I can be pretty stubborn when I have to be, so finally Jim took me back to our rig and we went to bed.

The next morning I couldn't even open my mouth. Jim called the security office and told them that he was taking me into Las Vegas to the hospital. Once we had dropped the rig at *Circus Circus' RV Park* in Vegas, we drove to *Sunrise Medical*, the nearest hospital.

The doctor, after looking at my swollen face, told me that my jaw was probably broken. Fortunately the x-rays showed no breaks, but it was severely sprained. He ordered pain medication, told me to eat soft foods or what I could suck down with a straw, and see my regular doctor as soon as I got home.

I didn't think I was ever going to open my mouth again, but we were still on vacation in Las Vegas and as long as I could walk we were still going to see a few sights. My appearance garnered more than a few askance looks from passers-by, but I ignored them. We went into the *Circus Circus* casino where there's an amusement park under the Big Top, and I managed to suck down some lunch at a buffet. The 'food' helped me feel a little stronger, so we continued to tour the Strip.

As we walked and enjoyed the sights, I noticed that my vision was a bit 'off.' At times it was like I was looking through water—you know, like when you're in a pool and you open your eyes underwater. Finally I mentioned it to Jim, but he said that my eyes appeared normal so we kept sightseeing for as long as I could.

Finally, I gave up. We returned to the rig before evening and that's where we stayed. When the huge fireworks celebration began, Jim and Audra went outside to watch while I remained in bed, my face so swollen that I looked like a chipmunk with its cheeks filled with nuts.

Still, I'm sure it was a happy New Year… somewhere.

It took us several days to get back to San Antonio. My determination and stubbornness didn't really help this time because I could only travel for a few hours before we had to stop. I was in a crimson haze of pain all the way home.

As soon as I could get into his office, Dr. J ordered an MRI of my head and face. I knew I had been badly injured, but I didn't know *how* badly. As it turned out, I had a broken right molar, a sprained jaw, two retinal hemorrhages, and a blown cervical disc at the C-6 and C-7. It's still hard to believe that all this damage occurred because one man was running to get a battery for his radio. He was a fairly tall man, and apparently when he hit me his shoulder clipped my jaw, which took the brunt of the impact.

Dr. J sent me to Dr. Karl Swann, a neurological surgeon, to evaluate my neck. My left arm was numb and I wasn't improving. Finally we decided that I needed surgery to correct the problems and to prevent permanent damage. Dr. Swann would go in through the front of my neck and install a titanium plate and four screws into my cervical spine. I'd spend two days in the hospital. It sounded simple enough, but the retinal bleeding took nine months to heal. The water that I thought I was looking through was actually blood collecting in my eyes. Finally my vision returned to normal, but I was a mess both physically and emotionally. Even though my family and friends were very supportive, I knew I had to rely on God to get me through this situation.

During this time in my life, I learned to be still with the Lord. He knew my circumstances and I just wanted to be safe at His feet while I prepared for this surgery. When the surgery was finished, Jim never left my side. Everything was successful and I returned home to heal.

Two weeks later I returned for a follow-up with Dr. Swann. Like most surgeons, he was very pleased with his handiwork. Of course I was too, and I was thrilled to be out of pain.

Half-joking, I said, "Since you did such a good job on my neck, I might let you look at my lower back someday."

He looked surprised. "What's wrong with your back?"

"Oh, it'll keep for now," I answered airily. "Don't worry about me. Today I feel pretty good."

I left his office and headed for the grocery store. Life was fine again.

𝄞

Throughout the school year, we study the Rand McNally Road Atlas and discuss where to go when school lets out for the summer. In the summer of 2003, Jim and I decided that we would make the big push up to Montana. There was so much that we wanted to see, and half the fun is getting there. *America the Beautiful:* It really is true.

We were thrilled when we crossed the border into Montana. Our first stop was the battlefield of Custer's Last Stand, located within the Crow Nation. From the top of a hill, as I gazed out over the magnificent rolling plains, I found it hard to believe this beautiful area had once been the site of such bloodshed and brutality. Markers signify each place that a soldier had died. It's very quiet here.

At the exit for the Custer Battlefield was a small casino, a church next to it, a few gas stations, and a log restaurant/gift shop filled with all the necessary touristy Indian and Custer stuff. We shopped for a little while, of course, and then headed north toward Billings, our first overnight stop in Montana. As we were driving down the highway, I spotted a large white tent out in a field with some workers nearby. I pointed to it.

"Look, Rank! They're going to have a Revival meeting!"

"It certainly looks that way."

I have no inhibitions when it comes to worship, and I love a good old-fashioned tent Revival meeting. There's something honest about coming together and praising the Lord with nothing but a canvas tent over your head and the good earth under your feet. There are no pretenses when you get saved in a tent Revival. Holy Ghost dancing stirs up the dust, so just spread a little straw around and dance, dance, dance all night!

Over our years together Jim and I have grown so much in the Lord, both individually and as a couple, that when we're on these long vacations together we find the Holy Spirit often speaks to us, and we know it's His voice. Maybe it's because we don't have the routine distractions of home: jobs, telephones, chores, computers, television. Also, there's nothing we enjoy more than spending time together. But on these trips we're alone with God, delighting in the world He created. Jim and I are very open with one another and we love to share what the Lord says to our hearts during these times. His Presence fills us to overflowing with peace and joy.

When we finally reached the Flathead Valley, called by some 'the gateway to Glacier National Park,' we never wanted to leave. I know it sounds trite, but this area truly is Heaven on Earth. The small towns of Kalispell, Whitefish and Bigfork are quaint as old postcards, and the pristine Flathead Lake is mirror-clear. The air smells so clean and sweet that I couldn't seem to breathe it in deeply enough. We decided to stay in this valley and explore all it had to offer.

Glacier National Park, located on the northwest corner of Montana along the spine of the Rocky Mountains, is the playground of the Lord. I've never been in a more beautiful place in my life. Television documentaries can't come close to depicting the true majesty and beauty of this area because the rarified atmosphere is more than something you see. It's also something you *feel*—and what you feel is indescribable.

We boarded a fully restored, open-topped bus that has shuttled up the mountains on the narrow, winding Going-to-the-Sun Road since the 1920's, and sat right behind the driver. As we drove into each switchback in the road, the scenery took our breath away. Waterfalls cascaded down from hundreds of feet above us at what seemed to be every corner, even splashing over the road itself, and I loved their picturesque titles: *Baring Falls, Weeping Wall,* and *Bird Woman Falls,* to name just a few. The driver pointed out various places of interest as we ascended into the mountainous region of the park. Finally, as we rounded a tight bend and gazed out over a picture-perfect meadow, we saw a craggy, slate-gray mountain in the distance. Our driver identified it as *Heaven's Peak.*

"Does anyone know why it's named *Heaven's Peak?*" he called out.

I couldn't restrain myself and bounced in my seat like a little kid. "I do! It's called *Heaven's Peak* because this is where God spends His summer!"

The other riders on the bus must have been politically correct because there was total silence, but I knew I was right.

Finally it was time to head back home, and once again we passed by the site of Custer's Battle in southern Montana. We had no plans to stop since we had been there earlier, but as we drove past, we noted that the large tent was still in place and a few people were milling around outside.

I glanced at Jim. "They're going to have church tonight."

"I think you're right."

Suddenly I felt the Holy Spirit speak to me. *Go back to the tent and pray for the wife of the pastor there. She's not feeling well.*

Without hesitation, I told Jim what the Spirit had said.

"Well, baby, if the Spirit told you we should go back and pray, turn this rig around and let's do it!"

I smiled and nodded. We drove for what seemed another five miles until we reached the next exit then headed back toward the tent.

Jim has always prayed for the sick and many times God has worked miracles through him. I've seen and experienced it myself. He is so filled with the Holy Spirit that James 5:16 in the Holy Scripture, which says that *the prayer of a righteous man availeth much,* has been manifested right before my eyes. One of my greatest privileges has been to stand at his side while he prays for someone else. I have often felt the heat and seen the glow that radiates from him during such prayers, and others have as well.

I've always known there was a calling on Jim's life. It was just a question of *when* God would reveal His purpose to him.

We pulled up to the tent in our rig and found a place to park easily enough, then climbed out and walked toward a few people who were coming to greet us.

"Are you the evangelists from Oklahoma we're waiting for?" one woman asked.

We shook our heads. "No," Jim answered. "We're just stopping in to visit the pastor and his wife."

The pastor's name, we discovered, was Buddy Rogers and he was a member of the Crow Nation. When we met, we shared with him the Word that the Holy Spirit had given us.

"My wife is Maria," Pastor Rogers answered, a little puzzled, "but I think she's fine. She's in the kitchen. Let me call her."

When Maria joined us, Jim asked, "Are you feeling all right, Mrs. Rogers?"

She frowned and shook her head. "Well, not really. I don't know what's wrong."

Although I'm sure that Maria and the gathering crowd were bewildered by our arrival, they accepted us without question and with genuine warmth. Jim prayed for Maria, anointing her with oil, and then a Crow man joined us, asking for prayer for his severe back pain, and then... before I knew it... something wonderful happened.

Tears began streaming down his face, Jim dropped to his knees in the dirt. "This is it! This is it! This is what God wants me to do!"

I felt the peace of certainty and nodded. "Yes, honey. It is."

Pastor Rogers put his hands on Jim's head and called down the blessings from God on His servant, a healer, the Holy Spirit had sent to them. At that moment we were all bathed and engulfed in the glory of God; we could hardly stop crying.

Jim had received his calling from the Lord, on land belonging to the Crow Nation, under the hands of a Native American man of God.

Pastor Rogers invited us to stay, but we declined. It wasn't yet our time. Still, we knew we would one day return to this place. We drove miles down the highway before Jim could speak. All he could do was look at me as the tears rolled down his cheeks. We both knew that our life-journey would never be the same again.

We spent many months in prayer, waiting to learn exactly what the Lord wanted to do with us. Our pastor counseled us as we shared the calling on our lives. We were a team, and we knew that whatever the Lord had for us, we were to do it together. We knew, without any doubt at all, that the Lord brought us together for a greater purpose, to serve Him with our whole hearts. The testimony of our relationship was a favorite among our friends and we loved to offer it, but we also knew that God had more for us to do in His kingdom.

As time passed, we knew that the Lord was teaching us and tuning us into His ways and His plan for our lives. I don't mean to preach, but sometimes, when you receive a calling from the Lord, it's very easy to get all fired up and enter the mission field before God has fully prepared you. People with the best and most honest intentions get ahead of God, then either burn out or become so arrogant that there's no room for what the Lord intended them to do in the first place. They often become their own god and serve their own worldly desires, all the while trying to cover it with a thin veil of holiness that true saints of God can see right through. We didn't want to fall into this trap.

God's ways are much higher than our own ways. His thoughts are greater than ours and His timing is perfect. We know that to wait on the Lord is our strength, and He will prepare us if we surrender completely to Him, to serve Him in a mighty way. The plans He has made for us are more wonderful than we could ever try to do on our own. So we wait, watch, and listen for His voice.

Jim continued to teach and I completed my coursework to become a certified appraiser of personal property. I had been a collector of art for many years, so I had a natural expertise as an appraiser of fine arts. I found that through my work as an appraiser, the Lord used me to share His grace and love with others. This is still true today.

God will take your talent and use it to His glory when you surrender your life to Him, and He will bless you at the same time. God is so good to those who love Him.

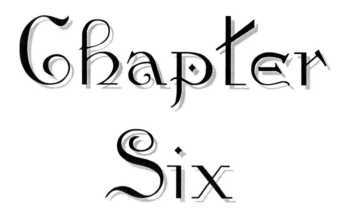

Chapter
Six

*He has made everything
beautiful in its time.*

Ecclesiastes 3:11

My life was puttering along very nicely when my world turned completely upside down. On September 30, 2004, Merck withdrew its medication Vioxx from the market, citing a study showing those who took the drug had an increased chance of heart attack or stroke. When I heard about it on the morning news, I couldn't believe my ears. I didn't care about some study and I didn't care about the FDA. I cared about being able to walk. I cared about being without pain. Every drug has side effects, some worse than others, but Vioxx had given my life back. To me, it was worth the risk.

I tried to reason with myself. *Maybe this is just a temporary recall. Too many people took that drug with no problems, so this has to be a fluke. Give it a little time and people will calm down. It will come back on the market.*

Reasoning didn't work. Finally, nearly hysterical with fear, I called Dr. J's office and reached his nurse. She was as upset as I was, but there was nothing they could do. They had been swamped with phone calls from other panicked patients, she told me, but their hands were completely tied. The ruling was final and the medication had been pulled.

Hanging up the phone, my heart thundered in my chest as I begged and pleaded with the Lord: *Please, please don't let this happen!*

I was so grateful for this medication and the quality of life it had given me, but I didn't have that much of it left and before long it would be gone. I cried all afternoon and by the time Jim came home, I was a complete mess. It was all I could do not to jump out of my skin the moment he walked in the door.

"What am I going to do, Rank? They took my Vioxx away! I need it to walk! How can they do this to me?"

He did his best to comfort me. "Maybe if we write Merck and tell them how well it works for you, they'll let you keep taking it. We could sign a release or something."

I appreciated his efforts, but all I could do was cry.

After Jim left for work the next morning, I sat at the kitchen table and had a big talk with Jesus. Over the years I'd taken many different medications for pain and I dreaded the thought of going back to them. They slowed me down and fogged me up. Nothing had helped me like Vioxx.

Finally, at the end of my rope, I came to the throne of the Almighty, threw myself down at His feet, and completely surrendered my bone disease to Him. Jesus would have to deal with this because I couldn't do it any longer.

When my Vioxx was gone, all I took in its place was Naprosyn, a fairly benign anti-inflammatory. As the days passed, I relied on Jesus more and more to keep me moving. He knew I had a family to care for and a career I loved. After all, I reminded myself, He had given them to me.

But I knew another spell would hit and I'd be stuck in bed again. I just didn't know *when*. Still, I refused to let fear rule my life. Every day became my personal walk in faith.

As the months passed, my pain increased and I tired more quickly, but I was still walking. I worked so hard to keep to my routine that even Dr. J was amazed. He was so concerned for me that when I went to see him he would just hug me tightly and assure me that if I needed him, he would be there. His support meant the world to me. It still does.

I knew that Dr. J had nearly run out of medications he could prescribe for me. I was very drug sensitive and many pharmaceuticals were on my allergy list. I could only handle so much. I knew he was frustrated because it was his job to help me and he was running out of options.

Dr. J was backed into a corner while this ticking time-bomb in my spine continued its countdown. He didn't know how long I had before I could no longer walk, but he never gave up. He was always there for me.

As I continued to battle spells of severe pain and partial paralysis, I was forced to periodically take to my bed once again. I was still able to get to the toilet with my walker, and Jim cared for me like a professional nurse. When I hurt I could see in his eyes that he hurt even more. I knew that if he could have taken my pain upon himself he would have done it, even though I would never have allowed him to do that. For whatever reason, this pain was mine and I continued to bear it.

In the summer of 2006 we decided to return to Montana. Since our first visit there a few years earlier, we had done nothing but talk about the beauty of the state and how we could hardly wait to go back again. It was like a magnet to my soul and I yearned to return. Since I felt that I was running out of time, we wanted to make Audra part of our Montana experience and decided she would fly out to join us there for a week.

To me, the decision to revisit Montana was an easy one, but Ronni, one of my closest friends, didn't seem to think so.

"Are you out of your mind?" she demanded. "What happens if you get up there and can't move? Rank *hates* to drive that rig, but he'll have to if you can't! Carolyn, there are hundreds of miles between hospitals! Honestly, sometimes I think you're the most stubborn fool God ever put on this planet."

"Ronni, you worry too much. If anything happens, Jim will take care of me. You know that. I trust him completely."

I knew her fears were well-founded and I even shared them to some degree, but I also knew that I had to do as much as I could before I couldn't do anything at all. I felt like I was racing the clock and I only had two choices: I could surrender or I could live. I intended to live.

This trip we took a different route straight up US Hwy 83, which took us through the plains. Of course we had to stop in Dodge City, Kansas, because I was a big fan of *Gunsmoke* and always watched the re-runs on television. We continued north to Nebraska and took a left turn in North Platte traveling west until we reached Wyoming. This route was easy and I really enjoyed driving across these states. The prairies were covered by an ocean of golden wheat fields and blue-green corn, and there was an abundance of unique birds. I even saw a magnificent male Golden Pheasant somewhere in Nebraska.

After we arrived in Montana we stayed a few nights in Billings, then took a northern road up through the high plains. We turned west about the middle of the state and drove to the well-preserved settlement of Lewistown, where we stopped for lunch and enjoyed a nice stroll on the square. The late Victorian-era city was a real gem and the people were small-town friendly. We could have spent a week or two in this sweet place, but our destination that day was Great Falls.

While we were in Great Falls, we visited the Charles Russell Museum. Russell was one of the greatest American artists to ever paint the west the way it really was. His depictions of Native Americans and their culture have been reproduced in books and countless other media. As a collector of fine art, I was aching to see this wonderful museum before I could no longer make such a long trip. I was thrilled to find that it was well worth our effort.

Another of our goals was to experience the eastern side of Glacier National Park, so we aimed for St. Mary, Montana. We stopped in the little town of Valier, where we had a terrific visit with Lame Bear, the proprietor of the *Medicine River Trading Company*, and his half-dozen cats. This place was a gold mine of authentic Native American clothing and artifacts, as well as western art by several well known artists. One of many great-grandsons of Comanche Chief Quanah Parker, Lame Bear thoroughly entertained us with stories about his lineage. Unable to resist its beauty, I purchased a hand-crafted medicine bag for Ronni, who was a student of Comanche Indian history.

The Blackfeet Indian Reservation borders Glacier National Park on the east. Grass-covered rolling hills and majestic snow-capped mountains in the distance give the eye so much to see that it's almost impossible to take it in. Still, I wanted to stop, sit quietly, and just *feel* the beauty of it all. A place like that is like a prayer without words.

As we continued on through the reservation toward St. Mary, I spotted a large animal running full speed through a field on our right, straight at us. At first I thought I was seeing things and took a second, harder look. We never see creatures like this in the city.

"Look, Rank," I breathed in awe, "it's a silver wolf!"

I slowed the rig down as the animal continued its pell-mell run toward the road. It paused for just a moment to look directly at us before it ran out in front of our rig, leaped over a fence on the other side of the road, raced up a hill and finally disappeared. I was speechless with wonder and my eyes filled with tears.

Surrounded as we were by Native American history, I was reminded that many indigenous people believe the wolf is a teacher, and when a wolf crosses our path we should remember we are all teachers to everyone we meet.

The eastern side of Glacier National Park is the most spectacular part of the park, and our camp in St. Mary allowed us to enjoy it all. The majestic mountains surrounding the area are indescribably beautiful, but the wind that whips and whistles off of them can be equally terrifying. The first night our rig rocked like a sailboat locked in an ocean storm and I really worried about whether or not the tent-campers nearby would survive, but the morning sunrise greeted a perfect day and I found that most of them had remained.

We traveled up into Canada to visit the Prince of Wales Chalet located on pristine Waterton Lake, one of the most photographed mountain lakes in North America. As I stood on an overlook taking my own pictures, I was filled with gratitude to God for letting me experience such a magnificent sight and giving me the stamina to continue on this incredible vacation.

We finally reached our primary campground in an area just north of Kalispell, a small town located in the heart of the Rocky Mountains, nestled in the northwest corner of Montana about an hour south of Canada. Here we would stay three weeks and Audra would join us. We had planned activities for every day that she was with us so that she could have the best Montana experience ever. When we picked her up at the airport, she burst through the door with tears of joy streaming down her face and I hugged her like I hadn't seen her in years. Finally, we were all together again—and in Montana, too! To us, this was as good as it could get.

For Jim's birthday, we decided to do something we had never done before: white water rafting. I had to do it… just in case. If I'm going to be paralyzed, I thought, it might as well happen while I'm having a good time.

We chose a 'medium difficulty' guided run on the Flathead River and I was seated in the middle of the raft. We were all outfitted with all the appropriate safety gear, and as we made our way onto the shuttle bus I said a prayer: *Okay, God, I know I shouldn't really do this, but I have to do it just once in my life. You know how it is.*

Throwing good sense to the wind, we were on our way down the river. The ride was thrilling and exhilarating and I'm glad I survived it; however, it will remain my first and last white water adventure. Jim and Audra can do it again someday if they want to, but my memories of this trip will be more than enough for me.

The week sped by and Audra returned to Texas by airplane. After she left we started to head south. Since forest fires were blazing throughout the southern part of the state, we laid out alternate routes as a precaution, but we really wanted to take the long way home. South of Billings the smoke from the fires grew thicker, scratching our throats and irritating our eyes, but we didn't stop. We drove on toward the Crow Agency, where we had seen the Revival tent a few years earlier. As we approached the exit for the Custer Battlefield, we noticed the tent had been erected in the field once again. We pulled into the parking lot.

My eyes burned from the smoke and I could hardly breathe, but we wanted to see Pastor Rogers if we could. After we learned he had had surgery and was unable to hold the Revival meeting that year, we found his home on the reservation. Because there was nowhere to park, Jim went inside to visit and pray for him while I stayed out in the rig in the middle of the street.

I was choking from the smoke and we had no choice but to get out of the area before we could stop for the day. The smoke didn't lift until we had crossed into Wyoming, and then it was replaced by the heat wave of the century. It was more than a hundred degrees at noon with no relief in sight, so we pulled into Douglas and stayed two days. My lungs needed to recover from the smoke and the heat didn't help. We decided that the safest thing for us to do was to drive at night.

When we finally drove into our driveway, we were exhausted but content. After only a few days in bed, I forgot my fatigue and scratchy throat. I was ready to load up and go back to the great Northwest. But I knew it was impossible.

God had given me a great gift, an opportunity to experience the world in a way many people only dream of, and I would be eternally grateful. I had been able visit museums and historical settlements and see magnificent panoramas that He had created with His own Hands, and He had allowed me to do it while I was standing on my own two feet.

He had heard my prayer and He had granted one of the most sincere wishes of my heart. But my world was in San Antonio, and I was ready to get back to it. Jim returned to school and I returned to my work.

Chapter

Seven

Keep me safe, O God, for in you I take refuge. I said to the Lord, "You are my Lord; apart from you I have no good thing."

Psalms 16:1, 2

I woke up at 3:00 in the morning on January 29, 2007 and knew something was wrong. I lay very still, hoping that the pain in my right side would go away, but it didn't. I had been in pain before, many times, but this pain was excruciating, launching in waves from my back to the middle of my right side. It was agony so fierce I could hardly breathe. I couldn't move.

Finally I reached over and woke Jim up. Yawning, he padded off to the bathroom to get me a pain pill and a glass of water. I lay in bed until morning.

As soon as his office opened, I called Dr. J and explained my situation. I don't know what I expected, but an order to go to the Emergency Room wasn't what I wanted to hear. Even when I was told that I could have a 'septic' hip, whatever that was, I refused to leave my house. I wasn't going to allow some sleep-deprived intern to fool with me, so I stayed in bed and suffered. I told you I was stubborn.

Audra was off that day and stayed with me while Jim went to work, arguing all the way out the door. When I still hadn't improved by the next day, I knew I was in trouble. I told Jim that I needed to go to the hospital, even though Dr. J was now out of town. Jim called Richard, a dear friend of ours who lived close by, and asked him to help get me downstairs and into the car.

By the time we reached the Nix Hospital, the pain was so intense my teeth were chattering and I couldn't stop shaking. They took me in right away, and I gave the attending physician my full history.

"It feels like I'm being stabbed with a Bowie knife," I gasped, "and they're twisting it around in there."

Now, if you're not a Texan and don't know what a 'Bowie knife' is, it's a pretty big knife. It was named for Jim Bowie who died defending the Alamo in 1836, and I was sure I was going to join him before the day was out.

The doctor ordered a CAT-scan of my hip area. A male nurse took Jim and me to Radiology. Once we were in an examining room and they tried to lift me out of the wheelchair to place me on the scan table, I emitted a bloodcurdling shriek that I'm sure the entire hospital heard. I went through that CAT-scan trembling uncontrollably, in so much pain that even hard labor couldn't match it.

Finally, the CAT-scan finished, we returned to the doctor, who ordered a heavy-duty steroidal drug via intravenous drip. I hate steroids and they don't like me much, either, but I knew I had no choice. Once they began to enter my body, I tingled all over and felt like I had ants crawling in my ears, but I knew it was the drug and didn't panic. Eventually my trembling ceased and the pain became bearable. The steroid didn't eliminate the pain entirely, but it did take the 'scream' out.

We returned home, where our friend Richard, a masseuse I had nicknamed *Little Brother*, was waiting with Audra. He helped Jim get me back upstairs, then took some of his lotions and began to message my legs and feet, which helped me to relax. I was so grateful he was there and that he was so supportive to my daughter.

My disease not only affected me but Audra as well, and it broke my heart because there was nothing I could do to prevent it. Since we have been through so much together, she and I are very close and my pain might as well have been hers. This is perhaps the most difficult aspect of any long-term condition: it affects everyone in the family without prejudice.

After I had spent a week in bed, Dr. J suggested that I go and see my rheumatologist. Dr. Winn hadn't seen me in years but gave me an appointment right away. He ordered a new MRI of my spine so we could see how advanced the bone disease had become. I was terrified.

I had been diagnosed with Degenerative Bone Disease when I was twenty-eight, and told that I would be in a wheelchair by the time I was thirty-five. Now I was forty-nine years old and I had fought this final conclusion with every ounce of strength I had. I had raised my child, continued to work, married the man I loved, and traveled the length and breadth of the United States. I had lived abundantly, subconsciously preparing for the day that this might happen. But now that day had arrived, and I still wasn't ready for it.

When the results came back, along with the radiologist's report, it wasn't good news. I immediately asked Dr. Winn if I should have surgery.

He shook his head slowly. "It's too risky, Carolyn."

I fought back tears. "Well, I need to do *something*, Dr. Winn! I'm having trouble controlling my bladder and my bowels now. I'm way too young to be having so many accidents!"

"I'm sorry, Carolyn. I see no choice here. We have to continue with pain management. Use *Depends* if you need them."

Well, I'm not one to take a single medical view and live or die by it. Where there's one opinion, there's going to be another one. I wasn't about to settle for pills and *Depends* at the ripe old age of forty-nine, so I took the report to Dr. J.

His response was immediate. "Carolyn, you need to call Dr. Swann and have him look at this. There's nothing else I can do for you and it's time to call in the big guns. Contact him and let's see what he says."

It didn't even occur to me to argue. As far as I was concerned, Dr. J was giving me a glimmer of hope.

The next morning I faxed the radiologist's report to Dr. Karl Swann, and not long after, his nurse Martha called me. "Carolyn, Dr. Swann has read the report and wants you in here right away. Bring your MRI films."

We decided that Jim and I would meet with Dr. Swann on March 13, 2007. I knew the situation was serious when I could get in to see the top Texas neurological surgeon in less than a week. I also knew I would make a decision that would affect the rest of my life.

𝄞

Jim and I sat quietly in one of Dr. Swann's examining rooms. With my MRI films in my hand, I walked to the window to admire the view from his sixth floor suite. Outside it was partly cloudy with a bit of springtime haze misting over the congested Medical Center area of San Antonio, but it was still beautiful to me. I was standing up to look out that window and I wanted nothing more than to keep standing.

Dr. Swann entered the room, gave me a hug, shook Jim's hand, and sat down. I gave him my films and kept my vigil at the window. He peered intently at the MRI films, then over to me, then back to the films again.

Finally he asked, "Do you have any pain?"

"Not right now, at this very moment. Nothing severe, anyway."

For some reason I remembered when he had first asked me to tell him about my back problems and I had refused to elaborate. He had repaired my neck following my accident at the casino, and I should have told him when he asked. But that was so like me, to just keep on going.

Dr. Swann interrupted my thoughts as he pointed to my films in the back-lit viewer. "Carolyn, you have some serious issues going on in your spinal lumbar region. How long have you been affected with this condition?"

I decided to sit down next to Jim while I explained my history to him. I wasn't going to conceal anything, this time.

"This is a very serious situation and I can't believe that you have endured this as long as you have. We need to operate as soon as possible. Your spine is unstable and any little shift could paralyze you permanently."

"How soon is soon?" I asked.

"No later than this week."

I stared at him in disbelief. "I can't do that!" I blurted. "We have to wait until school is out for the summer. I'll need help. I'll need Jim."

"That's too long, Carolyn! That much delay is too risky! Jim, when is school out?"

"The last of May—about two-and-a-half months from now."

I could see the frustration in Dr. Swann's eyes and I felt sorry for him, but there was nothing I could do about it. I wasn't doing this without Jim.

"Carolyn, I've already consulted my orthopedic surgeon, Dr. Robert Johnson, on your case. He agrees the urgency is real."

I shook my head firmly, my characteristic stubbornness setting in. "I won't do it until Jim can stay home with me."

Dr. Swann held up his hands. "Okay. I can see there's no sense in arguing. But if we have to wait until June—and mind you, I don't like it—we can make some preparations for this procedure."

Dr. Swann called his nurse to schedule the surgery and we all agreed on June 4, 2007. That bit of important business completed, he turned back to me. "Now listen to me carefully, Carolyn. When you go home, don't do anything that could cause your spine to shift. Don't clean house or even run the vacuum. Be very careful going up and down the stairs. Just take it easy, eat right and get plenty of rest.

"Also, Carolyn, since we have time, you can start banking your own blood at the blood bank. This is a very bloody operation and it's better if you have your own blood available."

The word *bloody* made this situation real and my heart gave a double-thump.

"I'll use the 'cell saver' to replace some of the blood loss as well," he continued. "You'll need to walk down the hall here and set an appointment with Dr. Johnson. When you meet with him at your appointment time, he'll go over the whole procedure. Do you have any questions?"

I shook my head silently and held on to Jim's hand like it was a lifeline, which in fact it was. We walked down the hall and set my appointment with Dr. Johnson, then made our way to the car. We sat quietly for a time as I pulled myself together.

The following week, I updated Dr. J on my visit with Dr. Swann, but Dr. Swann had already called him and told him about my upcoming surgery. Still, Dr. J listened and assured me I was doing the right thing. There are very few people that I trust completely, but Dr. J is one of them. He knew I had endured so many years of intense pain that I was out of options. Surgery was my last hope.

"This procedure is way too big for me to assist Dr. Swann," he told me, "but I'll be there. I promise."

The hard reality of my twenty-five-year struggle with this spine of mine was now front and center in my life. Time had finally run out for me, exactly as I had always known it would, and now I had made the one decision that could change my life.

But I had to come to grips with what I was about to experience if my family was to get through this. I had to be an example of strength and faith so that Audra could cope. She was still so young. I had to be of good courage for her sake, if not my own.

And so I prayed continually: *Lord, please help me. I need You to strengthen me and guide me on the journey I have before me. Amen.*

Ronni's mother, a tiny and frail woman more than eighty years old, went into the hospital for an aortic valve replacement. The night before her surgery, Jim and I went to visit and pray with her. She looked so small; I don't believe she weighed ninety pounds at the time. As Jim kneeled down and prayed, anointing her with oil, I felt the Lord's gentle Presence moving all around us. I knew with peaceful certainty she would come through the surgery safely.

"Trust in the Lord," I told her softly. "God is good, and He'll take care of you."

Then, as we left the hospital, I heard the Spirit whisper to my own heart. *Carolyn, will you trust Me to take care of you?*

April was a month of prayer for me. I spent each day alone at home, sitting in my favorite chair in our family room. I had been reading my Bible daily first thing in the morning for many years, but now I spent more time in His word. I often listened to our local radio station KDRY, an all-teaching Christian radio station, and heard my favorite programs during the day.

With orders from my doctor not to do much of anything, I spent my day sitting quietly at my desk or in my chair, waiting for the time when I could begin fixing dinner for my family. I stopped doing much around the house, as Dr. Swann had requested, but cooking for my family was an absolute *must* for me. I was able to do the dishes without too much risk to my spine, but I could do little else. I felt a bit useless, but Jim and Audra took over without complaint whenever they could.

The dust built up on the furniture, the floors needed sweeping, and I probably should have named the animal hairballs accumulating in the corners, but I ignored it all. For the first time in my life, I learned to let go and just *be*.

On May 1, 2007 I met Dr. Robert G. Johnson, Dr. Swann's orthopedic surgeon. He's much smaller than Dr. Swann and his manner is much different, but I liked him. Audra had joined Jim and me for this visit, and I realized she was circling her own emotional wagons in preparation for this newest phase in her life.

Dr. Johnson looked intently at the MRI films. "It looks like this disease has affected your L2 through S1 vertebra, and I believe that your L1 is in the early stages of degeneration."

I stopped him. "May I ask you a personal question?"

"Of course."

"Do you believe in God, Dr. Johnson?"

He turned away from the films and met my gaze head-on. "I do. I believe."

I smiled and nodded. "Good. Because if you didn't, I couldn't let you touch me no matter what."

"I understand, Carolyn. I respect your faith. I truly believe this surgery will help you."

Audra spoke up in a small, trembling voice. "Could my mother be paralyzed during this, Dr. Johnson?"

He didn't shy away from the question. "That's always a possibility, of course, but I'm going to do everything in my power to keep that from happening."

Now was the time for me to step in and make my desires known, desires I had thought about and prayed over, long and hard.

"If you get in there, Dr. Johnson, and you find there's no hope for success, I want you to cut whatever nerves need to be cut so I'm without pain. I can live in a wheelchair just fine, as long as I don't have pain."

Dr. Johnson said nothing. He just looked at me intently for a long moment then answered, "That statement alone tells me how much you need this surgery. We're going to take good care of you. We'll do our very best, I promise."

I stood up and hugged him. When he left the room, his nurse joined us and showed me the type of hardware that would be installed to secure my spine. When she departed, my little family held each other and tears streamed down my face.

This is really going to happen to me, to us. This isn't a bad dream. This is reality.

Still, I knew that our faith in the Lord would hold us together, no matter the outcome. We were a family and we lived in God's Grace.

We left the room and walked to the reception desk, where Dr. Johnson was talking to a nurse. He looked over at me and lifted a finger in greeting. "Oh, by the way, Carolyn," he said. "Remember to start banking your blood. This is a very bloody procedure. You have the forms, right?"

I gulped and nodded as he walked away to see his next patient. *Bloody.* There was that word again. Once more reality crashed right into me.

I hadn't noticed a petite, pretty woman about my age waiting at the counter until she spoke softly, "Don't worry, honey. Everything will be fine."

There was something so peaceful about her; a special glow emanated from her that was strangely soothing. Curious, I took a step toward her.

"What's your name?"

"Linda."

"Have you had surgery?"

"I have, and my life is so much better now."

I swallowed hard. "I'm going in on June 4th for a 6-level construct. I think that's what they call it."

Linda smiled. "June 4th is my birthday. I'll remember to pray for you that morning."

"Would you really? Are you a Christian?"

"I am."

I couldn't help myself. It was an automatic reaction that simply felt right and imperative. I took this mysterious woman in my arms and held her close.

"I'm a child of the King, too," I whispered.

She returned my embrace then took a step backward. Her face was radiant. "I see the Presence of the Holy Spirit upon you. You'll be fine."

Before I could answer, the nurse called my name and I moved back to the counter. While I answered her questions, I looked over my shoulder for Linda…but she was gone.

I searched for her in the parking lot so I could thank her for her comfort, but I never saw her again.

To this day, I wonder if she was really a patient—or an angel sent by God.

Chapter Eight

But David said to Saul, "Your servant has been keeping his father's sheep. When a lion or a bear came and carried off a sheep from the flock, I went after it and rescued the sheep from its mouth. When it turned on me, I seized it by its hair, struck it and killed it. Your servant has killed both the lion and the bear; this uncircumcised Philistine will be like one of them, because he has defied the armies of the living God. The Lord, who delivered me from the paw of the lion and the paw of the bear will deliver me from the hand of this Philistine.

1 Samuel 17:34-37

I had a month to get my affairs in order before the surgery. I updated my will, and took Jim and Audra into my office to show them where all my important papers were located. I wanted them to be prepared to step into my shoes immediately if they had to.

The doctors said I would be in recovery for at least eighteen months, so that also required planning. Jim would be my main source of help, but he needed to be relieved once in a while. Audra had to step up and do more of the housework. She had her regular chores and worked full time, but now there would be so much more to do.

There are only the three of us in this little family unit. All our relatives have passed away, but God has given us some really wonderful friends. I knew I could lean on them during the healing months.

Every day I spent quiet time in prayer. I sat in my chair and spoke with the Lord as if He were on the couch across from me. I don't know any other way to speak with Jesus. I know He is King of kings and Lord over all, but I communicate with Him like He is my best and most intimate friend—because He is. No one knows me better than Jesus. Even though we can conceal our feelings from people, we can hide nothing from Him. He knows all about us.

I found that being completely open and honest with the Lord was wonderful for the soul. I just poured out my heart and He listened to me. My relationship with Jesus had reached a level of trust I had never known, and I rested in His peace and love.

Jim and I were seeking a new church family during this time. We had been members of a little country church located near the small town of Fayetteville, Texas for about eighteen months, where Jim had been the associate pastor. We had attended faithfully, even though the church was nearly 125 miles from our house, but finally the ever-increasing price of gas forced us to leave and look closer to home.

Every Sunday we tried a new church, only to be disappointed with the content of the service or the character of the leadership. Many pastors have their own agendas, which have nothing to do with God's plan for the people. Today the organized church seems to have so little to do with God and so much more to do with the world. Many churches no longer even serve the Lord's Supper, and often pastors preach without the use of a Bible in the pulpit. This baffles me. Maybe I'm just old school, but I need more than music and dancing and a few happy thoughts.

I want the true Word of God!

One day while in prayer, I told the Lord I had to call the blood bank and start the process for saving my own blood for surgery. God knows how I hate needles, and having my blood drawn for even the simplest test is very stressful to me, so I asked Him to give me the nerve to do what I needed to do.

But then, as I was struggling to gather all my courage and make that phone call, I felt the Spirit of the Lord speak to me, as He had so many times before.

I don't need your blood. Just rest.

When I told Ronni of my decision not to have my blood drawn, her reaction was fairly typical of any sane person, I'm sure, and I understood it.

"Carolyn, how do you know this isn't just wishful thinking on your part? How do you know *God* is telling you this? It could just be what you want to hear. I think you ought to have it drawn and saved, just in case. How hard can it be? I really don't think God will hold it against you."

But, as usual, I dug in. "It's not necessary. I'll be fine."

I didn't know what Dr. Swann would think, but I did know the Lord had spoken. No matter what anyone else thought, I trusted His Word.

♪

On May 30, 2007 I went to see Dr. J, hoping to have a few minutes alone with him before my surgery. As we visited in his office I remembered how he had always done his best to ease my pain; my journey over the years had never been a solo one. Dr. Greg Jackson had always been there for me, and with me.

"I'll do everything I can to be at the hospital Monday morning," he assured me, "but if I can't make it, I'll be calling the surgical team periodically. Don't worry about a thing, Carolyn. These doctors are the best."

At that moment I loved him so much and felt such a surge of gratitude that I had to give him a huge hug. My tears stained his shirt, but he hugged me right back.

The morning of May 31st, during my quiet time with the Lord, I began to recall Bible stories, specifically those depicting great acts of faith and courage: David, Moses, Elijah, Paul... I suppose each of us can find someone in the Bible with whom we can identify, in both the Old and New Testaments. I've always felt that temperamentally I was more like Peter of the New Testament, but that I had lived the life of Joseph in the Old Testament. Peter was bold and quick to speak; so am I. Joseph was rejected then abandoned by his family and finally exiled to a distant land, where he struggled with poverty, abuse, and loneliness. The same happened to me. Yet both these men survived their circumstances and moved forward in their lives, always attempting to serve the Lord.

I have tried to do this as well. But on this particular morning I felt more like a young David thrust in the midst of Saul's army. Even though David had no armor and wasn't trained to fight with a spear or sword, he knew God was with him. I understood—and shared the fear I was certain David must have felt as he met the Philistine giant who had slaughtered all of Saul's best fighters. Tears of dread pricked my eyes and I began to pray.

Jesus, I'm going up against my Goliath in a few days and I need your strength. There's nothing I can do but trust in You. I pray that whatever the outcome of this surgery is, it will be Your will for my life. I surrender it all to you, Lord."

And then, in a hushed voice that soothed the panic in my heart, the Lord's words were clear and definite: *Carolyn, the battle is mine. But get your rocks.*

At first I thought my fear had pushed me right over the edge. *Rocks! What rocks?* But then I remembered: David had chosen five smooth stones to take with him to face Goliath that day. With only a slingshot and those five smooth stones, he would face the most colossal warrior in the world. But David was certain of his victory. He knew the Lord was with him.

I eased myself out of my chair, walked outside to my back driveway, and began to look for my first smooth stone. When I found it, I reached down, picked it up and called, "I found one today, Jesus!" Then I came back into the house, put the stone in a sandwich bag, and carefully placed it on my Bible.

In a strange twist of fate, I realized I had five days before my surgery: I would collect one stone each morning and add it to the bag.

On Saturday morning Audra asked curiously, "Mom, what are these three rocks for?"

"Those are mine, Audra. Don't worry about it."

She didn't ask me again.

Sunday morning, after I had collected my fourth stone, Jim and I drove to the east side of San Antonio to attend services at the Greater Evangelist Temple. Although we still hadn't found a new permanent church home, we had shared in their Watch Night service on New Year's Eve and thoroughly enjoyed it. I wanted to worship somewhere I had been before.

A warm and cloudless morning reminded me that summer was fast approaching, so I dressed comfortably in a lightweight skirt and blouse. A few members recalled us from earlier and welcomed us back, but everyone was friendly whether they remembered us or not.

After we sat in seats located about midway in the sanctuary, I placed my bag of stones on my lap and held Jim's hand tightly. The music was filled with praise and worship, and I absorbed it deep into my soul. Since this was First Sunday, they served communion in their traditional manner, and the pastor, Reverend Clem Steward, brought forth a powerful message straight out of the Bible. As he preached, many *Amens!* and *Go Ahead Ons!* enthusiastically punctuated his sermon. I like this kind of interactive church stuff; it feels personal to me.

When Reverend Steward finished his message he turned away from the pulpit to take his seat, but then he halted. I was surprised when he walked back to the microphone and looked around the congregation for several moments, a puzzled frown on his face. Finally he asked, "Is there someone here with back problems?"

My hand shot straight in the air and I managed to pull myself up. "It's me, Pastor, it's me!" Tears began to flow.

When Pastor Steward motioned for me to come to the front of the sanctuary, Jim and I walked together. I leaned heavily on his arm but I was unaware of pain. Instead I cried and praised Jesus all the way down that aisle; I could feel Him all around me. When Jim shared with the congregation that I would have serious back surgery the next morning, Pastor Steward asked that his Elders and the church Mother join us so that they could all pray for me. As they gathered around me and lifted their voices, I felt a rush of warmth suffuse my entire body. An indescribable peace entered my spirit.

The peace that passeth all understanding...

The Lord had met me, face to face, in the hour of my greatest need.

That night we went to bed early because we had to be at the hospital at 4:30 in the morning, and I actually slept. I was able to rest before the most stressful medical event of my life. If that isn't the power of the Lord, I don't know what is! Before we left the house, I found my fifth rock, put it in my little plastic bag, and carried it with me to the hospital.

The atmosphere in the surgical waiting room at the Methodist Hospital was thick with anxiety. As the minutes ticked by, I watched more and more patients and family members enter through the swinging doors, their faces etched with fear and worry. I reached for Jim's hand and held it tightly.

"I wish I could give these folks some of the peace I'm feeling," I said softly. But I knew I couldn't, so I prayed for them silently. When I heard my name called, I followed a nurse into a small room where she gave me a gown, some tight stockings to help ward off blood clots in my legs, and told me to put my hair up in what looked like a paper shower cap. That was it. I was all dressed up and ready to go.

Not long after, I was wheeled down to the surgical prep area where someone inserted an intravenous drip in my arm. The nurses moved quickly and easily between patients as if they were all participating in a familiar dance routine. Jim stayed close to me and I clutched my bag of rocks.

God is with me, for the battle is the Lord's...

A hospital chaplain came in to offer prayer and words of encouragement to all the patients, but when she stopped by my bed she looked surprised. "I don't think there's anything I can say to you this morning," she told me with a smile. "You look fine and fresh as can be."

I smiled back. "The Lord is responsible for how I look, but I thank you coming by."

She nodded and moved to the next bed.

Next my anesthesiologist came in and introduced himself. "I'm Dr. Gerald O'Gorman. I just have a few questions."

When we were finished with his interrogation, I squeezed his hand. "Don't you lose me, Doc. I have too much to live for."

Dr. O'Gorman reassured me with a pat on my shoulder. "I have no intention of losing you, Carolyn." And he left me as quickly as he had appeared.

Then Dr. Johnson stopped beside my bed. He looked from Jim to me. "Are you ready to go?"

I nodded.

"Any questions?"

I shook my head.

"Okay. This surgery should take about six hours. I'll send

word out to you every once in awhile about how she's doing, Jim. But don't worry. Everything will be just fine."

"Dr. Johnson," I said softly, suddenly a little worried, "I didn't bank my blood."

He grinned. "It's okay. You're Type-O positive and we have four bags on order for you." He patted my foot and walked away.

Finally Dr. Swann joined us and gave me a hug. "Are you ready, Carolyn?"

"I am. And I've got my rocks."

He looked startled, like he wasn't sure he had heard me correctly. "Rocks? What rocks?"

"These are my faith rocks, Doc. I'm going up against my Goliath, so I thought I'd better get my rocks for battle." I pulled my bag of rocks out from under the sheet and handed it to him. "Here, Dr. Swann. You keep these for me. When this is over, you can give them back."

Dr. Swann met my eyes and gave a solemn nod. Then he slipped my bag of five smooth stones into the pocket of his white lab coat.

Chapter Nine

*The seventh angel sounded his trumpet,
and there were loud voices in Heaven, which
said: The kingdom of the world has
become the Kingdom of our Lord
and of His Christ and
He will reign for ever and ever.*

Revelation 11:15

I hear familiar voices. Someone is holding my hand.

Why are they talking about food?

I'm hot, and thirsty.

Why can't I move?

I can't open my eyes. Someone rubs my arm. It's a soft hand, a gentle touch. I manage to speak. "I'm hot."

"I'll get you a damp cloth."

The cloth feels wonderful, cool on my forehead. That's

much better.

They're still talking about food. Are they hungry? Why don't they eat? I'm so thirsty!

I still can't open my eyes, but now I recognize a voice. It's Audra. She sounds scared. "Mama? Mama, can you hear me?"

I can't answer, but I recognize another, huskier voice. It's Ronni. "She's coming around now, sweetie. Give her a little time."

Why is Ronni here? Where am I?

I hear Jim, and my friend Lula...

Why do they keep talking about food?

I have to tell them. They need to know. I struggle to raise my head. I hear my own voice. It sounds very loud, but that's okay. This is important.

"The best jailhouse food is in Norman, Oklahoma," I announce.

Ronni's laugh throbs with relief. "Well, we know where *she* is right now."

"Mama, move your feet."

What?

"Mama, please! Wiggle your toes, please!"

I move my feet and wiggle my toes and Audra actually laughs so hard she snorts. I understand. A single tear slides down my cheek. The surgery is finished... I can move...

I'm alive! Praise Jesus, I'm alive!

It was in the late afternoon before I could speak and answer a few simple questions. After the nurse had adjusted my bed and tubing, then showed me how to use my call button, she left the room. As the door whished closed behind her, Jim sat next to me and took my hand.

"How are you, honey?"

"Okay, I guess. A little foggy. Did everything come out alright?"

He kissed my forehead. "We're better than alright. We've had a miracle, honey. Even the doctors are stunned by what happened. But you just rest and I'll tell you all about it later."

"Daddy, please don't leave me," I whispered, using one of my favorite terms of endearment for him, and gripped his hand even more tightly. I was terrified to be alone, call button or not.

"I'm not going anywhere, honey. They've already set up a bed for me and everything."

"Tell me about my miracle."

"Are you sure? You're not too groggy?"

I shook my head. "Not for that. Tell me."

"Well, after your surgery was finished, Dr. Swann and Dr. Johnson came into the waiting area where we were all camped out. They were shaking their heads, which scared me at first. But then, as they got closer, I saw they were smiling so I knew it was all right."

"What was it?"

"Well, this is what Dr. Swann said: 'Thirty years of surgery between us and we've never seen anything like this. This is a very bloody surgery, but Carolyn lost less than half a glassful.' Ronni and Audra both broke down and cried with relief, you know, but I really wasn't all that surprised." He kissed the top of my hand and grinned at me. "I mean, after all, I've never known you to do *anything* the way other people do it."

When I read my surgery report much later, I saw that the doctors estimated my blood loss to be around 250cc. Not bad for a procedure where they wanted me to reserve at least two pints of my own blood. My incision didn't even bruise.

But, like Jim, I wasn't surprised. After all, I figure that if God could hold back the Red Sea for Moses and the Israelites, He could hold back the tide of my own blood to help the doctors...not to mention, me.

Very early the next morning, Dr. Swann came in to check on me. I opened one bleary eye to see him standing at the foot of my bed. A tall, slim man with short sandy hair and wire-rimmed glasses, Dr. Swann really didn't look like the champion I felt he was. He was the only doctor I had ever seen who hadn't been afraid to take the risk of repairing my spine, and I owed him so much.

Dr. Swann put the sandwich bag with my five smooth stones on the table beside my bed and glanced at my chart.

"How was your night?"

I managed a groggy smile and tried to focus. "I lived, Doc."

"Well, that's a good thing, don't you think?"

I nodded then asked the question at the forefront of my mind. "Did you find a mess in there?"

"I sure did, Carolyn. But we opened the canals that the nerves pass through, and stabilized your spine. We put in two titanium plates and installed twelve screws, so I think you'll have less pain now. Airport security is going to go nuts for the rest of your life, but the truth is, everything went better than I expected."

"Well, you had my faith rocks, Doc," I reminded him. "God did a mighty thing for us."

Dr. Swann just smiled and nodded. "Indeed He did." He

looked more closely at my chart. "We're going to get you out of bed today."

"Today? You're kidding!"

"Nope, not kidding. That's the plan."

I grabbed my little bag of stones and held them close to my chest.

Man, am I going to need these rocks today! I've got tubes coming out of everywhere and they're going to make me walk! Why not just go ahead and ask me to do the Texas Two-Step? That's just as crazy.

But I didn't argue aloud. He was the doctor, and he was the best. I trusted him with everything I had.

Suddenly I had an idea. "Dr. Swann, do you have any faith rocks of your own?"

He shook his head. "No, I've never even *seen* any faith rocks before you shared yours with me."

I held the plastic bag toward him. "Well, here then. I want you to have mine. You *need* faith rocks, Dr. Swann. You never know when you'll face Goliath in your life. Use them as your weapon."

Dr. Swann took the bag of stones from me and looked at it for a moment. Then, smiling thoughtfully, he slipped it into his pocket. "Patients have given me a lot of different things over the years, Carolyn, but this is a first. I'll keep them, I promise."

I nodded sleepily, and my answer jumbled crazily through my mind without a beginning or an end. I thought I said it aloud, but I wasn't sure…

And you won't ever forget me, either, will you, Doc? Or that God guided your hand and held back my blood…You're a wonderful doctor, but God was with you.

As Dr. Swann walked away from my bed, I heard the stones clicking against one another in his pocket and smiled softly. I closed my eyes and slept.

♪

Well, the nurses did return, and they did get me out of bed. I shook like a newborn foal from my head to my feet, but I made it. I used a walker, of course, but I managed to take one step forward then another, and when they asked me to take a step to the side, I was able to do that, too. And then I actually took a few steps backward to the bed. My teeth chattered and I trembled from the shock of it all, but I made it. And, like a marathon runner who has just managed to pull himself across the Finish Line of a 50-mile race, I was exhilarated.

God is good. God is so good. Thank you, Lord!

A couple of days passed and my appetite began to return. I wanted some fruit. Hospital food no longer cut it for me, even though it didn't seem to bother Jim in the least, and I was getting frantic for some real sustenance.

"Daddy, would you go down to the cafeteria and see if they have any fresh fruit? I really, really want some fresh fruit."

As always, Jim accepted his mission without complaint. He put his ever-present book on the window ledge and headed for the door.

Alone in my room for the first time since my surgery, I thought about all we had experienced over the last two days. The hospital staff had been wonderful to us, even allowing Jim to put an air mattress on the floor so he could sleep more comfortably. The catheter was still in my bladder, which wasn't pleasant, but it was certainly manageable. The important thing was that I had stood up on my own yesterday, and I could rotate my feet. Now I slowly raised my knees a bit just to see if I could do it. I could, and without much pain.

Closing my eyes, I took a deep breath and released it in pure relief. *Thank you, God, for bringing me through this. You are so merciful and so good to me; I don't deserve this. It's only Your Grace, Father.*

Jim entered the room, carrying a bowl of strawberries that looked so good my mouth immediately began to water. As soon as I had eaten them I felt stronger and more aware of my surroundings. I looked around my room. There sure seemed to be a lot of 'stuff' out of order.

"Daddy, could you maybe straighten up a little bit? I might have some company today."

He chuckled. "If the clutter is bothering you, I know you're on the mend."

I smiled back then wrinkled my nose in distaste. "Something smells funny in here. Can you smell it?"

"A little bit. Maybe it's disinfectant..."

Jim emptied the trash, and the staff came to clean the room, but the smell lingered.

I tried to ignore the odor and ate my lunch when it arrived. Then, somewhere in the far, far distance, I heard the faint notes of what seemed to be gospel music. It was playing on a radio, or maybe it was a CD. I didn't know where it was coming from, but it was pretty. Frowning, I turned off the television and looked around the room.

"Daddy, do you hear that?"

Jim looked up from his book. "Hear what?"

"I think someone is playing a radio next door."

He shook his head. "I don't hear anything. Is it bothering you?"

"No, I'm just trying to hear what's playing."

"Well, let me go out and see where it might be coming from." Jim left the room but returned a few minutes later, a perplexed expression on his face. "No, no music out there that I can hear."

"Well, I hear it from *somewhere*," I insisted. "At least they have it on a gospel channel."

"They're doing some construction upstairs. Maybe you're hearing their radio."

I tried not to laugh, finding it hard to believe that construction workers would be playing gospel music. "Maybe," I said aloud.

Just then the nurses, who were exceptionally sensitive to my condition, arrived to drag me out of bed again. After I had taken a few deep breaths to prepare for the marathon ahead, they pulled me up to a sitting position on the side of the bed. After a few more minutes I gripped my walker and, using all the strength I had, managed to haul myself to my feet. I don't believe I've ever been so determined to walk. With a helper on either side of me, I made it all the way to the door and out into the hall. Then I turned around and headed back into my room.

One of my helpers egged me on like a high school cheerleader. "You go, girl! Wow, would you look at that! Just aim for that bed, honey!"

I shook my head. "No, I want to sit in that chair."

"Are you sure?"

"Yes. I want to sit in that chair."

"Okay, honey, let's go."

I heard clapping as I managed to sit down, but I think it was Jim. I didn't need all this encouragement. What I really needed was to bathe. That foul odor was following me everywhere I went, and I had had enough.

"I want a shower."

"Not a chance," one of the nurses objected. "You've got a catheter and you can't get your incision wet."

As usual, I dug in. "Listen," I said firmly, "something stinks in this room and I think it's me. If you'll just get me something to cover this incision, I'll be fine. Jim will help me."

The nurse knew there wasn't much point in arguing, and I appreciated that she didn't waste my time. I was going to take a shower if it killed me.

Finally, bathed and under clean sheets, I closed my eyes to sleep. And somewhere in the far, far distance playing very softly, was the music.

𝄞

We discovered that what was producing such a hideous smell was my catheter, which in turn had caused a disgusting bladder infection. The nurses immediately cleaned me out and put me on strong antibiotics. It wasn't long before the odor was gone and I was feeling better.

I could still hear the music but now it was growing louder, and sometimes I thought I heard lyrics. It still seemed like it was coming from somewhere in my room, but Jim swore he couldn't hear a thing. I touched the table in front of me to see if it vibrated, but it didn't.

Still, the music came in more and more clearly, steadily building in perfect synchronization and tone. I couldn't tell if it was inside my head, outside of it, or just filling the room from some unseen source. Then, as I listened more closely, I slowly came to realize that this was choral music without any accompaniment. There were no instruments—no harps or pianos or organs; just tens of thousands of flawless voices singing in superb harmony.

I looked at my husband anxiously. "Daddy, you don't think that Dr. Swann left his I-pod in my back during the surgery, do you? Maybe that's why I hear this music and you don't!"

Jim laughed out loud. "I don't think so, honey, but you can ask him the next time he comes in."

So I did, almost the moment he walked into my room.

"Dr. Swann, do you hear music playing?"

Shaking his head, he glanced up from my medical chart. "No, I don't hear anything. Why?"

"Oh…I don't know. I was just wondering…"

Now, I know that stress can play tricks on your mind. I've been a victim of it, just like everyone else has. But this incredible music was *real*, as if I was sitting in a heavenly theater absorbing the towering voices of ten thousand angels. That music gradually enfolded me in warmth and peace and love. But I didn't know where it was coming from.

"Daddy, I'm not losing my mind. Seriously, I can hear this music."

Finally Jim sat beside me on the bed and took my hand. "Honey, I believe you. But maybe this music isn't for anyone but you. Don't worry about it. Just enjoy it."

The next day Jim and I made our way around the entire ninth floor of the hospital. Gripping my walker as I shuffled down the hall, I saw other patients lying in their beds, some obviously in a great deal of pain. As I passed their rooms, I said a silent prayer for each of them.

Father, please bless them like you've blessed me. Please comfort them and give them peace.

When I finally made it back into my bed, I closed my

eyes in utter exhaustion. Once more that marvelous music enfolded me in a silken cocoon and bathed me in warmth. Pure voices in this angelic choir harmonized perfectly in what I began to recognize as old hymns, creating the most exquisite music I had ever heard. As I listened, marveling at the peace I felt, I began to recognize a few words—words of praise and adoration for the Lord.

Finally, no longer caring where it was coming from, or whether or not anyone else heard it, I let go of myself and floated into the music.

Chapter Ten

Then Jacob made a vow, saying, "If God will be with me and will watch over me on this journey so that I return safely to my father's house, then the LORD will be my God..."

Genesis 28:20, 21

When I was finally released from the hospital on Saturday afternoon, I went home wearing a large brace, like a hard plastic corset, to protect my spine. Even though Jim did his best to avoid the ever-growing San Antonio potholes and smaller bumps on the road, every jerk and jolt jarred my entire body and sent waves of pain crashing through me. But I survived the ride. When we finally pulled into the driveway, I viewed my beloved Victorian home through a haze of grateful tears.

Our house was built in 1890 and I've lived here for over

thirty years. I've put my heart and soul into this house, decorating it with as much historical accuracy as I possibly could, and I believed that I would recuperate better here than anywhere else in the world. Set back from the street, it's shaded by a canopy of native pecan trees and looks warm and reassuring. I love to sit on our large front porch with all our 'outside' cats and watch the birds splashing around in the birdbath. I'm very secure here.

Still, the steps leading up to the porch were only the beginning of an enormous feat for me. I had yet to climb upstairs to the second level of the house and into our bedroom.

Many of my friends had suggested that I stay in a hospital bed downstairs during my recovery and bypass the stair issue entirely, but I wouldn't have it. I wanted to live like a normal human being and sleep in my own bed. Because I knew what was best for me, I wouldn't listen to what other people called 'reason' and refused to change my mind. I was determined to climb up my grand staircase and get into my big plantation bed if it was the last thing I ever did.

I managed a smile and feeble wave for Richard, who was standing in the driveway awaiting our arrival. Jim slowly pulled me out of the car and Richard supported me while I adjusted the walker. I said a silent prayer, took a deep breath, and then started toward the steps. One foot in front of the other, inch by excruciating inch. When I reached the front porch, Jim moved the walker so that I could lift my foot to the first of four steps. It felt like it had taken years to get this far, but I finally made it up the steps, across the wide porch, and into the house. Jim helped me into an antique throne chair we have in our foyer.

"You rest here, honey, and we'll unpack the car."

I certainly wasn't going to argue. Exhausted, I leaned my head back and closed my eyes, trying to catch my breath, and felt the soft fur of my cat as he rubbed against my ankles. I patted my lap.

"Come up here, Butter," I murmured. "Come see Mother."

Like all cats, Butter is inordinately curious, so he jumped into my lap, purring loudly, and began to check me out. He pushed his cold nose against my neck, and investigated my back brace, and all but inhaled my skin as he attempted to isolate all the strange smells I had brought home with me. I knew that he completely understood I had been through something major and survived.

Then, for some reason, it really hit me for the first time. I was home, and I was in one piece. *I was going to have a life.* My eyes flew open and filled. As tears streamed down my cheeks, I thought I was going to burst with joy. My gratitude was so deep and fervent that I couldn't contain it. I lifted my hands towards heaven and raised my voice in a completely inadequate but heartfelt prayer of thanksgiving.

"Oh, thank you, Jesus! Bless your name! Thank you, Lord, thank you! Hallelujah!"

And then, there it was, home with me: The music. Oh, my, I can still hear the music! That heavenly choir filled with thousands of perfect voices resounded and rang through our entire house, filling my spirit with ecstasy. I caught my breath in delight.

When Jim entered the foyer carrying my bags, I looked at him, my face awash in tears of pure elation. I held my hand out to him.

"Daddy, the music came home with me. I can't believe it. It came home with me."

He smiled and took my hand. "Then you know it's for you, honey. It's a gift from God."

Oh, how I wish he could hear it, too!

But he couldn't, and he was right. It was a gift from God.

Finally, with Jim and Richard's support, I began the long climb up the staircase, holding tightly to the banister. Each step seemed as high and insurmountable as the side of a sheer cliff, but I felt God's strength moving in waves all around me, like a protective shield. And then, just when I thought I couldn't take another step, I saw the bedroom door and called out to Jesus in thanksgiving once more.

I was going to make it.

🎼

Richard, my dear friend and *Little Brother*, is a confirmed bachelor in his fifties, and he'll make someone a good wife if he ever grows up. There's not much he can't do. He cooks, cleans, repairs and installs, plants, mows, paints and, to top it all off, he's a licensed massage therapist.

Little Brother stepped in and did anything I needed, from caring for my little dog while I was in the hospital to helping Jim and Audra. He helped me to manage my pain through massage, something I had never really experienced before. I trusted him, which meant more to me than anything else. God has given us such good friends.

After a few days, Jim and Audra had established a routine for my care and comfort. Jim took care of all the heavy stuff like pulling me up out of bed, taking me to the bathroom, giving me a daily shower, and dressing me in a clean gown. He took those wedding vows '*In sickness and in health*' to a whole new level.

Audra did the laundry, shopped, cleaned, and relieved Jim whenever she could. Little Brother cooked meals and brought them over to us, and helped me with exercises that focused on strengthening my legs. He was wonderful.

Our friends didn't forget us once I came home, and their love and support helped us so much. Sometimes, in the evening, a bunch of them crowded into the bedroom to visit. I loved to roll on my side so I could show them my incision, just like any proud patient. A formidable cut ran all the way from where my bra strap usually lies down to where the good Lord split me, if you know what I mean. My incision still hadn't bruised but was closed on the surface with surgical staples. It was like someone had installed a big zipper right down the center of my back.

I didn't go downstairs for about ten days, until I returned to the doctor to have my staples removed. As time passed I continued to regain my strength and felt more like a younger, healthier form of myself every day. I had no doubt that I had done the right thing by having the surgery.

I knew I would be several weeks in bed, so I began to crochet an afghan for Dr. Swann. I found it pretty easy to crochet lying down, and Jim began to read me the epic book *Roots* by Alex Haley. My husband has an excellent voice and many of our friends think he should be on the radio, but what they don't know is how animated he can be. He can read a book so that the characters jump right out of the pages.

Consequently, I was entertained no matter how long I had to lie in that bed. But my greatest comfort was the wonderful music that only I could hear. It never completely ceased. Only the volume level fluctuated, depending on what I was doing. If Jim was reading to me, the music was soft, like a low radio in the next room. When I was alone, I closed my eyes as the music swelled and filled my room, as if I were seated in a heavenly cathedral being ministered to by my own personal choir of angels.

Every day, as I rested in this magnificent music, I began to focus on words that were gradually becoming clear to me. And I noticed that now there was a single instrument accompanying this chorale music, although I had no idea what it was. But, at times between the songs, there would be a long silence followed by the long steady tone of a great horn. Then, sometimes, the horn would sound three times and the choir would burst into song again. I had played the trombone in concert band when I was in junior high school, but I had never heard this horned instrument before in my life. It was pure and soft and even in pitch.

Whenever I heard this tone, I knew the choir would begin its great repertoire again. The words to some of the songs were familiar, but the melody wasn't. For example, the words to *Amazing Grace* were the same but the tempo was different. I recognized *How Great Thou Art*, but the tune was different and some unfamiliar words added. Then there were the indescribably glorious songs I had never heard before.

I knew I had to find a way to record this experience in my memory. "Daddy," I said one evening, "could you write down some of these words I'm hearing?"

Nodding, Jim opened a notebook lying beside him and began writing the words as I repeated them: *His healing blood, it covers me. His wondrous love, it strengthens me.*

The music completely covered every inch of my being, as if I had dived into the deep end of a heated pool, and I felt as if I was floating softly somewhere between this world and heaven. I was embraced and engulfed in the essence of these pure angelic voices. I continued to pass on to Jim the Spirit's partial interpretation of the lyrics as I received it:

His Love and Glory covers me
Bow down before Him—adore Him
I lift Him up and sing my song
Wonderful love
He's worthy of all
And from His Glory...
Holy Spirit

Oh, look and see—the shelter is there
Kneel down before Him
His Blood that heals us
His Love, eternally...

I didn't know how it was happening, but I knew what I was hearing was real.

Epilogue

*I will give you praise in the great assembly;
among throngs of people I will praise you.*

Psalm 35:18

After only two weeks had passed, I said, "Rank, I need to go back to that church tomorrow, okay? I need to let them know I made it through, and I want to tell them about the miracle God gave me during surgery."

As always, Jim agreed. I think of all the many blessings the Lord has given me, Jim Rankin is the greatest.

"Well, if you think you're up to going," he said with a smile, "I'll get you there."

We had ordered a large rolling walker with a seat, which I used when I went to get my staples removed, and it was a lifesaver. It supported me when I needed to navigate and gave me a place to rest as well. I still had to wear my brace, too, of course, so I looked like a mobile advertisement for rehab items whenever I went out, but I didn't care. I was going to church, no matter what.

Sunday morning, Jim awakened me early with a bit of breakfast and then helped me to the shower. I selected a dress my brace would fit over without restricting me too much, and Audra styled my hair. Finally I was ready to go. After all we had been through, the Rankin family went back to church together, a walking testimony to the Grace of our Lord Jesus Christ.

Heads turned as we made our way up the aisle to find a seat. A lady usher with a big smile pointed me toward a place up front where I wouldn't violate the city's fire code by blocking access to an exit. But the fire in the church that morning wasn't smoke and ash. It was the fire of the Holy Spirit as His presence filled the church.

The pastor gave me the microphone and asked me to testify what the Lord had done, and boy, I just let it go. I had to tell it—what the Lord had done for me and my family, how he held my blood back so the doctors could operate for hours on my spine, how I got up and walked the entire ninth floor of the hospital on the third day. God used the whole surgical experience for His glory and I was free from 25 years of pain. There wasn't a dry eye in the church.

As folks shouted out to the glory of the Lord, I heard later that people had been healed of back pain and other medical conditions right then and there. There was dancing and singing in the Spirit as the blessings of the Lord moved over His people. I was so blessed by the love of the Saints that we now have joined the fellowship of Greater Evangelist Temple Church of God in Christ.

Doctors Swann and Johnson had told me that I would need to go to rehab after the surgery, but that never happened. The Lord was my rehab. Four weeks after coming home, I was out and about, calling on clients again. I used the walker, then two canes, and then only one cane for a few months. And ever since I put that one cane away, I've had no need for any assistance or support to get around. Dr. Johnson continued to see me at three-month intervals and just shook his head in amazement at the speed and full extent of my recovery.

"Are you doing the exercises in the booklet I gave you?" he asked at one of our appointments.

I shook my head, grinned, and looked him in the eye. "Doc, it's just God doing a great thing in me, that's all."

Finally the music began to slowly fade away, but it lived with me for at least four weeks. I deeply miss hearing the heavenly voices of that great mass choir. It brought me such comfort and peace that I can never thank the Lord enough. The music was one of the greatest blessings of my life.

Ten months after my surgery, Jim and Audra had a birthday party for me. It was my *Fifty and Fabulous* party, and all my friends came out to celebrate with us. I showed off my x-rays so everyone could see (and admire) the hardware that held my spine together, and everyone had a wonderful time. There was so much love in the restaurant that night that even the wait staff was moved to tears at the end of the party.

I hit the big Five-O in a grand way, not the least of which was that I stood before my family and friends on my own two feet. From the depths of my soul, I thank Jesus for all His blessings.

But that wasn't the end of the music.

In October 2008, Jim and I went to a nearby church to hear a talk by Sid Roth, a Messianic Jewish evangelist speaker and writer whom we admire. At the meeting a man stood up and began to blow an enormous animal's horn. I'd never seen or heard anything like this, but it emitted the same sound I'd heard between the songs of the heavenly choir when I experienced the music.

I learned later that this ancient instrument, known by devout Jews as a *Shofar*, was made from the curved horn of a ram or other kosher animal. But once I heard that long, steady sound at the meeting, I knew in my heart that the music had come straight from heaven, a gift of healing from Jesus for me.

I'm so humbled to have received such a blessing, and to know that God has a purpose for each of us if we only surrender our will to Him. Just as He poured his Grace over me in the form of heavenly healing music, He will make a way for you, no matter what you're facing, if you let Him into your life.

This may be the 21st Century, but God is still in the miracle business—today and forever. I'm living proof of it.

THE END

Glossary
&
Documentation

Spondylosis: Immobility and consolidation of a vertebral joint.

Lumbar Radiculopathy: Disease of the nerve roots in the lumbar section of the spinal column (lowest five vertebrae).

Decompressive Laminectomy: Removal of the posterior arch of a vertebra in order to relieve pressure on (decompress) the spinal cord.

Stenosis: Narrowing of an opening in the body.

Facet Arthropathy: Disease of the small plane surface (facet) of a vertebral joint.

Orthotics: A term for devices or procedures designed to restore or improve function, usually in joints.

Sagittal Alignment: Alignment along the sagittal (head to toe) plane of the body.

Debridement: Removal of foreign or dead tissue until healthy tissue is exposed.

Transverse Process: Projections on the right and left (transverse plane) of the vertebra.

Capsule: Structure enclosing the disc between vertebrae.

Exude: To ooze out.

Synovial Cyst: A sac found in joints.

Cancellous Bone: Bone in a lattice-like structure.

Cancellous Aggregate: Lattice-like material massed or clumped together.

Morselized: In this context, bone in particle form.

Neural Foramen: An opening or passage for nerves.

Interbody Fusions: Joining of two bodies into one; in this case, vertebrae.

Pars: A division or part.

Decorticated: Removal of portions of the outer covering of a part.

Lordosis: Forward curvature of the lumbar section of the spinal column.

Osteocel: Bone repair product containing stem cells.

Surgicel: Blood clot inducing material.

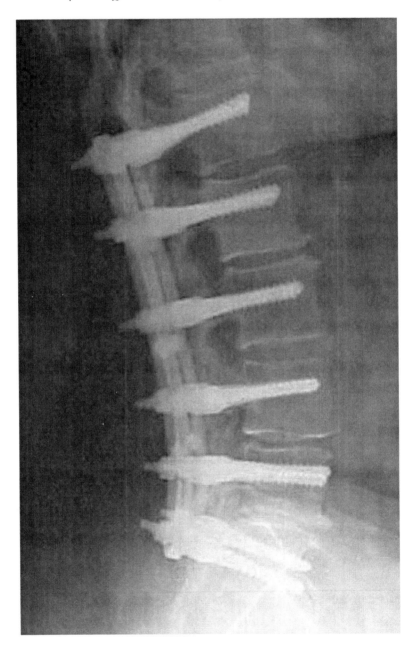

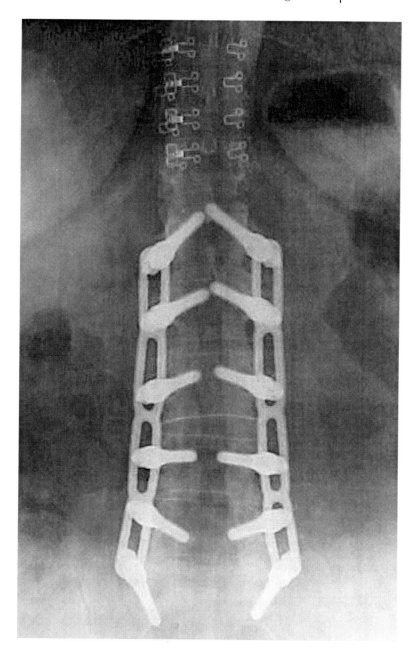

SOUTHWEST TEXAS METHODIST HOSPITAL
METHODIST CHILDREN'S HOSPITAL OF SOUTH TEXAS
7700 FLOYD CURL DRIVE
SAN ANTONIO, TX 78229

PATIENT'S NAME: HUEBNER-RANKIN, CAROLYN S
DOB: ~~~~~~~~~ AGE: 49 SEX: F
ATTENDING PHYS: Dr. Karl W Swann

UNIT NO: K00809876
ACCOUNT NO: W119532198
PT TYPE: ADM IN
ROOM NO: H.982

DATE OF ADMISSION: 06/04/07
DATE OF DISCHARGE:

DATE OF OPERATION: 06/04/07

PREOPERATIVE DIAGNOSIS:
1. Degenerative disk disease, lumbar.
2. Facet arthropathy with lumbar radiculopathy.

POSTOPERATIVE DIAGNOSIS/IMPRESSION:
1. Degenerative disk disease, lumbar.
2. Facet arthropathy with lumbar radiculopathy.

OPERATION/PROCEDURE PERFORMED:
1. L1 to sacrum posterolateral fusion.
2. L1 to sacrum internal fixation with the ROC-plate system.
3. Bone graft, local, plus stem cell harvest, bilateral iliac crest.

SURGEON: Dr. Robert G. Johnson
ASSISTANT: Dr. Swann
ANESTHESIA: General anesthesia.
ANESTHESIOLOGIST: Dr. Gerald O'Gorman

SPECIMEN REMOVED: None.

ESTIMATED BLOOD LOSS: 250 cc with none replaced.

HISTORY: This pleasant lady had been seen preoperatively at the request of Dr. Swann with a complaint of severe back and leg pain unresponsive to conservative measures. X-rays showed degenerative changes at multiple levels. MRI scanning confirmed this with loss of signal on the T2 weighted images and narrowing of the disks from L1 down to and including the L5-S1. She had facet arthropathy. She had neural foraminal stenosis. It was elected to proceed with a decompression and fusion from L2 down to the sacrum.

DESCRIPTION OF FINDINGS/TECHNIQUE: General anesthetic with endotracheal intubation was administered. A Foley catheter inserted. The patient was placed prone on the Fisk frame. The back was prepped and draped in the usual manner. A standard midline lumbar incision was made, paravertebral muscles were stripped, and intraoperative

OPERATIVE REPORT

Robert G Johnson
4410 Medical Dr., #610
San Antonio, TX 78229

PATIENT NAME: HUEBNER-RANKIN, CAROLYN S   ACCOUNT #: W119532198

Dictating Physician's copy / STATUS: Draft   Page 1 of 3

SOUTHWEST TEXAS METHODIST HOSPITAL
METHODIST CHILDREN'S HOSPITAL OF SOUTH TEXAS
7700 FLOYD CURL DRIVE
SAN ANTONIO, TX 78229

PATIENT'S NAME: HUEBNER-RANKIN, CAROLYN S
DOB: ~~~~~~~ AGE: 49 SEX: F
ATTENDING PHYS: Dr. Karl W Swann

UNIT NO: W00809876
ACCOUNT NO: W119532198
PT TYPE: ADM IN
ROOM NO: H.982

DATE OF ADMISSION: 06/04/07
DATE OF DISCHARGE:

x-ray was taken to ascertain the correct level and sagittal alignment.
The lateral structures were debrided of soft tissue and muscle
attachments including the transverse processes of L1 through L5, ala
of the sacrum, lateral portions of the pars, and the facet joints.
Lateral gutters were packed with sponges. The pathologic findings
included facet arthropathy with hypertrophy, irregular facets, poorly
defined capsule with exuding synovial cystic material at multiple
levels. Bone marrow was now harvested, a total of 240 cc split
between the two iliac crests. The bone marrow was processed by the
fusionary method for stem cell concentration. The stem cells were
added to crushed cancellous bone to form a stem cell cancellous
aggregate. In addition to this, there was a moderate amount of local
bone which had been derived from the posterior elements, debrided of
soft tissue, and morselized. At this point, a decompression was
carried out including a laminectomy at L1-2, down to and including
L5-S1. Pathologic findings included some central stenosis and neural
foraminal stenosis. The decompression is the subject of a separate
report by Dr. Karl Swann. The bone quality was good. I did not feel
that interbody fusions would add anything to the contrast. The
lateral structures were decorticated with a Midas Rex bur and this
included the transverse processes of L1 through L5, the ala of the
sacrum, lateral portions of the pars and facets with an AM-8 type bur.
The facets were decorticated in preparation for a facet fusion. The
pedicles of L1 through S1 were identified with the gearshift probe,
tapped with a 5.5 tap, and into each pedicle was inserted an 8+
ROC-screw measuring 7 diameter by 40 length in the lumbar pedicles and
7 by 36 in the sacral pedicles. The purchase was good. Two plates
measuring four slots were bent to the appropriate degree of lordosis.
Bone graft was packed into the lateral gutters and the facet joints.
I supplemented the bone graft with 10 cc of Osteocel. The plates were
then secured to the screws with acorn nuts and tightened to
approximately 80 to 100 inch pounds with the side handle wrench. This
gave a rigid construct. The level above moved normally.
Intraoperative x-ray showed good position of the screws and good
sagittal alignment. The midline was rechecked, reprobed, and covered
with fibrillar Surgicel. A deep Hemovac drain was left in place. The
deep layer was closed with interrupted #1 Vicryl, 2-0 subcutaneous,
and staples in the skin, followed by a sterile dressing.
OPERATIVE REPORT

Robert G Johnson
4410 Medical Dr., #610
San Antonio, TX 78229

PATIENT NAME: HUEBNER-RANKIN, CAROLYN S   ACCOUNT #: W119532198

SOUTHWEST TEXAS METHODIST HOSPITAL
METHODIST CHILDREN'S HOSPITAL OF SOUTH TEXAS
7700 FLOYD CURL DRIVE
SAN ANTONIO, TX 78229

PATIENT'S NAME: HUEBNER-RANKIN,CAROLYN S
DOB: ~~~~~~~~~ AGE: 49   SEX: F
ATTENDING PHYS: Dr. Karl W Swann

UNIT NO: W00809876
ACCOUNT NO: W119532198
PT TYPE: ADM IN
ROOM NO: H.982

DATE OF ADMISSION: 06/04/07
DATE OF DISCHARGE:

At the start of the procedure, appropriate antibiotics were given
intravenously. Throughout the procedure, the wound was frequently
irrigated with bacitracin solution. The Pulsavac with three liters of
saline and one amp of GU antibiotic. Estimated blood loss was 250 cc.
Cell Saver was utilized, but insufficient blood was harvested to
reinfuse. Sponge and instrument counts were correct. The patient was
returned to the recovery room in satisfactory condition.

Job #2403049

_____

Dr. Robert G Johnson

JOHROG ,KLB
dd: 06/04/07 1226
dt: 06/04/07 1343
cpcs rpt#: 0604-0208
cc: Dr.

OPERATIVE REPORT

Robert G Johnson
4410 Medical Dr., #610
San Antonio, TX 78229

PATIENT NAME: HUEBNER-RANKIN,CAROLYN S   ACCOUNT #: W119532198

Dictating Physician's copy / STATUS: Draft   Page 3 of 3

SOUTHWEST TEXAS METHODIST HOSPITAL
METHODIST CHILDREN'S HOSPITAL OF SOUTH TEXAS
7700 FLOYD CURL DRIVE
SAN ANTONIO, TX 78229

PATIENT'S NAME: HUEBNER RANKIN, CAROLYN S
DOB: ████████   AGE: 49   SEX: F
ATTENDING PHYS: Dr. Earl N Swann

UNIT NO: 900809896
ACCOUNT NO: W119532198
PT TYPE: ADM IN
ROOM NO: H.582

DATE OF ADMISSION: 06/04/07
DATE OF DISCHARGE:

DATE OF OPERATION: 06/04/07.

PREOPERATIVE DIAGNOSIS: Lumbar spondylosis with radiculopathy.

POSTOPERATIVE DIAGNOSIS/IMPRESSION: Lumbar spondylosis with
                                       radiculopathy.

OPERATION/PROCEDURE PERFORMED: Decompressive laminectomies
                                  L1,2,3, 4 and 5 bilateral
                                  partial medial facetectomies
                                  and bilateral foraminotomies.
                                  L1-2, L2-3, L3-4, L4-5 and
                                  L5-S1.

SURGEON: Dr. Earl N Swann.
ASSISTANT: Dr. Robert O. Johnson.
ANESTHESIOLOGIST: Dr. Gerald O'Gorman.
ANESTHESIA: General endotracheal.

COMPLICATIONS: None.

TRANSFUSIONS: None.

SPECIMEN REMOVED: None.

ESTIMATED BLOOD LOSS: 250 cc for total procedure.

DRAINS: Hemovac.

DESCRIPTION OF FINDINGS/TECHNIQUE: The patient was taken to the
operating room where a general endotracheal anesthesia was induced.
Intravenous antibiotics were administered preoperatively. A Foley
catheter was inserted into the bladder. She was carefully placed into
the prone position on the laminectomy frame with all pressure points
appropriately padded.

The lumbosacral region was shaved, prepped, and draped in the standard
sterile fashion. A midline linear incision was utilized. Using sharp
                      OPERATIVE REPORT

Earl N Swann
4410 Medical Dr #610
San Antonio, TX 78229

PATIENT NAME: HUEBNER-RANKIN, CAROLYN S   ACCOUNT #: W119532198

Dictating Physician's copy / STATUS: Draft   Page 1 of 3

SOUTHWEST TEXAS METHODIST HOSPITAL
METHODIST CHILDREN'S HOSPITAL OF SOUTH TEXAS
7700 FLOYD CURL DRIVE
SAN ANTONIO, TX 78229

PATIENT'S NAME: HUEBNER-RANKIN,CAROLYN S
DOB: ~~~~~~ AGE: 49 SEX: F
ATTENDING PHYS: Dr. Karl W Swann

UNIT NO: W00809876
ACCOUNT NO: W119532198
PT TYPE: ADM IN
ROOM NO: D.992

DATE OF ADMISSION: 06/04/07
DATE OF DISCHARGE:

dissection, the dissection was carried down through the subcutaneous
tissue and fascia.

Using subperiosteal dissection, a bilateral exposure was made. The
intraoperative x-ray was utilized for precise anatomic localization.
Self retaining retractors were introduced. Laminectomies were
performed at L5, 4, 3, 2 and 1 with bilateral partial medial
facetectomies and bilateral foraminotomies L1-2, L2-3, L3-4, L4-5,
L5-S1, all utilizing thin lipped Kerrison rongeurs. There was central
and lateral recess stenosis at each level due to a combination of
ligamentum flavum thickening, facet arthropathy and spondylosis. The
above maneuvers dealt with this very nicely, however and following the
decompressive procedure performed, we could pass a blunt tipped
uterine sound out along each nerve root into the neuroforamen
bilaterally indicating excellent decompression.

We carefully inspected the disks at each level. They bulged somewhat.
There was, however, no frank extrusion or significant compression of
the thecal sac following the decompressive procedures performed.
Although bilateral partial medial facetectomies were performed, facet
integrity was preserved throughout the procedure and the intraspinous
connection between T12 and L1 was preserved as well for stability.

Next, Dr. Robert G. Johnson performed a bilateral lateral fusion and
internal fixation with my assistance. The details of this portion of
the procedure will be dictated in a separate note by him. It should
be noted that following placement of graft material and hardware, the
nerve roots were rechecked and remained nicely decompressed.

Next, meticulous hemostasis was achieved. The wound was copiously
irrigated with antibiotic solution. A drain was placed in the
subfascial space and brought out through a separate stab incision.
The wound was closed in layers using interrupted #1 Vicryl for the
fascia, interrupted 2-0 Vicryl for the subcuticular stitch and skin
staples. We were told that all sponge, needle and paddie counts were
correct. Sterile dressings were applied. The patient was taken to
the surgical recovery room in good condition, having tolerated the
procedure well.

OPERATIVE REPORT

Karl W Swann
4410 Medical Dr #610
San Antonio, TX 78229

PATIENT NAME: HUEBNER-RANKIN,CAROLYN S   ACCOUNT #: W119532198

LaVergne, TN USA
02 August 2010
191733LV00003B/38/P